Diet

Food Units

Milk	Fats	Fruits	Vegetables	Soups
4	3	3	3	5 a Week
348	155	175		

Calorie Allowance: **1800**

Milk	Fats	Fruits	Vegetables	Soups
4½	3	3	3	5 a Week
392	155	175		

Calorie Allowance: **2200**

Measures by Volume

1 quart = 4 cups

1 cup = 8 fluid ounces — it could weigh anything on scales within reason of course

1 oz. = 2 tablespoons

1 tablespoon = 3 teaspoons

16 tablespoons = One cup

GROWING UP SLIM

GROWING UP SLIM

BY
POLLY BOLIAN

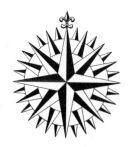

AMERICAN HERITAGE PRESS

NEW YORK

Library of Congress Catalog Card Number: 70-111658
07-006380-X

TABLE OF CONTENTS

1592826

V

GROWING UP SLIM

To Catch a Rabbit

So you have a weight problem—or think you have. You want to do something about it, and you've tried a half-dozen schemes. You've read the articles and believed the glowing promises.

Maybe you've tried the macrobiotic diet, and you're as devastated as a flooded rice paddy. Or you've made a monkey of yourself with the banana and skimmed-milk routine. By now, you're crashed out and getting the picture: it's tough, joyless, and it doesn't work—for long. That extra padding is still there plus a few more pounds for company.

Well, what now?

The first thing you do is cheer up! Behind that gloomy cloud of tasteless food and starvation dieting is a bit of silver lining. The experts have turned up some very interesting facts about fat—how it gets there and why.

And they know a lot about YOU and your overweight problems.

You aren't alone. Millions of American teen-agers have the same problem. All share certain traits in common. And all share certain types of experiences that may be decisive factors in weight gain.

Perhaps you're a "young" overweight. You've just started fretting about the pounds. Or maybe you're an "old" overweight, and you've been lugging excess padding most of your life. Either way, you want to get it off and keep it off.

Although this book is intended primarily for those with a

1

serious weight problem, anyone can adapt the plan to fit his own needs. In these pages, you will find a *basic system* for battling the bulges along with a variety of techniques to boost your batting average. And you will come up with some ideas and techniques of your own.

But most important of all, you will learn some startling facts about fat that will knock a lot of myths and folklore into the well-known cocked hat.

Keep Your Chins Up!

Overweight isn't just a matter of weighing too much. Neither is it a matter of overeating. As world-famous nutrition authority Dr. Jean Mayer points out, "To say that obesity is caused by overeating is like saying that alcoholism is caused by overdrinking."

Many complex things may cause obesity. Some are beginning to be understood; others remain a mystery.

Experts know, for instance, that your emotions are as much involved as your physical body. Overweight affects your moods, attitudes, judgment, and behavior. It affects the way you feel about yourself and the way you feel about others. And all of these things, in turn, affect your weight!

Yes, it does sound a little like chicken-or-egg. But scientists have found important clues in the way you feel about yourself. They've also found some pretty important clues in the way the world feels about *you*. These and other findings are going to help you solve your weight problems.

In and Out of a Pinch

As in the old recipe for making rabbit stew, "First catch the rabbit." In this case, your first ingredient is the problem. Are you really overweight? What makes you think so?

Perhaps it would be fairer if we put it this way: are you really over*fat?* There's a basic difference between the two, particularly with teen-agers.

How do you spot the fat that spells overweight?

Don't reach for the weight tables. You may be overweight according to the tables, but if that extra weight is solid bone and muscle, you aren't over*fat!* Therein lies the difference.

Likewise, you could be slightly underweight, by the tables, and still be overfat.

Take a look at the line-up of the Green Bay Packers. Now, there's a hard-rock wall of finely honed athletes. But nearly all of them would qualify—by height to weight comparison—as being overweight.

Confusing? The problem is really simple. There is so much variation in body build, in distribution of fat, and in actual body fat content, that it's almost impossible to design a "desirable" weight table with any sense to it.

Attempts have been made to classify height to weight relationships by small, medium, and large frames. This is of no help to a growing teen-ager. What you want to know is whether or not you're *overfat*. Weight tables can't reveal *actual body fat*.

So what's the answer? The fat content for each individual skeletal and muscular structure can be measured scientifically. But for practical purposes, we will use the following Pinch Test, recommended by the National Research Council:

> With your arm hanging down in a relaxed position, find the exact midpoint between the top of your shoulder and your elbow, on the backside of the arm (the triceps muscle).

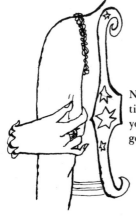

> Now, gently pinch up a fold of skin and fat tissue. Don't pick up the muscle with it. If your skin fold is over an inch thick, it's a good bet you are, in fact, over*fat*.

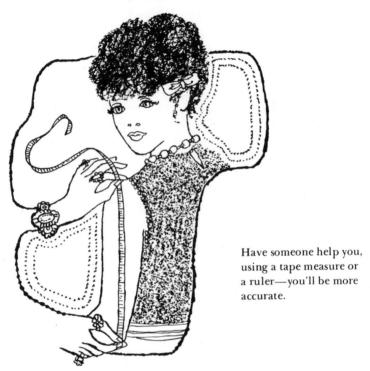

Have someone help you,
using a tape measure or
a ruler—you'll be more
accurate.

If you're still in doubt, do the same test on a fold of skin
just below your shoulder blade, several inches to the right or
left of your spine.

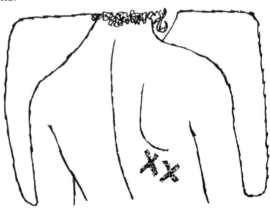

Why is the Pinch Test a better guide? Because the relationship of skin-fold thickness to body fat, at these two spots, is independent of height or build.

Mirror, Mirror?

Yes, you can look in the mirror and decide you're fat. But that brings up another important point in judging your overweight—your expectations, or how you "see" yourself.

Many teen-agers think of themselves as being fat. Very often this self-image is completely unrealistic, particularly when teen-agers go through the "puppy fat" stage. Or when they think they should match the "fashion model" ideal.

For boys, the puppy fat stage usually begins around twelve or thirteen years (but not always. Each is an individual, remember.). Girls are, as a rule, fatter than boys, but the puppy fat stage shows up somewhat earlier. They aren't always over*fat,* however, and that's what you're trying to judge.

During your teen years, your body and emotions are subject to intense and sudden changes. But growth spurts don't all happen at the same time and in the same way to everyone.

Girls may develop wider hips, adding more bone and muscle weight. Yet, in height and other measurements they may take time to catch up.

Boys may fill out, then suddenly grow taller, or vice versa.

All of which is just another way of saying: take a close, realistic look at yourself in terms of your age, your growth and development, your body build, and your expectations before you make a final judgment. You may not need a weight program at all. You may only need a bit of patience.

In the words of one expert, "Unless the fat is visibly excessive and persistent over too long a period of time, there is no cause for alarm." This should be the yardstick with which you catch your rabbit.

2

TUNING IN THE PICTURE

Okay, so you really fit the bill. The Pinch Test tells you that you're overfat. And the fat *is* excessive and persistent. You've got to lose weight.

But hang in there a moment. This could be the most important decision of your life. There are still two ingredients we haven't mentioned yet.

So let's tune in the rest of the picture.

We've talked about one area of the overweight problem —the body. Two others are equally important. *Any* problem that deeply affects you must include

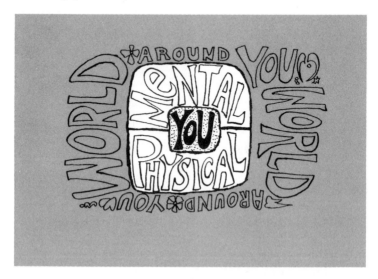

You can't separate the physical from the mental. And you can't ignore the world around you. The three are as inseparable as Siamese triplets (if there is such a thing!). Each one directly affects the other.

Before you make a decision to change your life, you need to know the whole scene.

Fair Weather and Foul

Not too many years ago, the plump look was very much in style. An extra twenty pounds meant health and wealth. Plumpness was proof that one did not have to do manual labor (thus working off excess pounds).

Then, machines took over the tough, backbreaking jobs. As the nation moved swiftly into a scientific and technological revolution, two things happened. We began producing (and eating!) an abundance of rich foods. But we grew less physically active at both work and play.

Before we knew it, we were a nation of spectators sitting on our ever-broadening *derrières* watching others carry the ball. Fatness was no longer a mark of distinction. Overweight became a national health problem.

Soon the message was loud and clear: thin is in, fat is out.

Hundreds of books and articles were written, solemnly assuring us the answer was simple: lower the calories, control the appetite. We were told that fat couldn't be blamed on glands, or hormones, or "metabolism." The overweight ones just had no "will power." They were merely weak and self-indulgent.

Society keeps the pressure on. The overweight are made to feel guilty about their excess pounds. Since the answer is simply a matter of self-control, the fat man is letting himself go, not "doing something about himself." This is "bad."

A Crown of Scorns

Does it all sound a bit moralistic? You bet it does! Never in history has a nation had such punitive and moralistic attitudes toward obesity. Fat is equated with sin, and the fat ones are an easy target. The normal-weights feel pretty smug and superior—after all, *they* have "will power."

Even the psychologists and psychiatrists voice the same attitude in another way. As Dr. Mayer points out, "they are adding fuel to the moralistic fire when they say obesity is due to neurotic or emotional problems—again, a flaw of character."

To claim that some kind of "character flaw" causes obesity puts the cart before the horse. Some experts believe this view is naive in light of new research into the complex workings of the body chemistry. Attitudes, emotions, reactions, feelings, personality traits, should be seen as a *result,* not a *cause,* of obesity.

This theory puts overweight in its proper framework since it relates to many recently discovered physical and genetic processes. It also challenges society to change its smug assumptions and re-examine its moralistic attitudes.

Dr. Mayer and other experts have recognized that the overweight in our society constitute a minority group that suffers prejudice and discrimination at every level. This discrimination takes the form of very real pressures that help to create and prolong the problems of the overweight.

There are many other theories. But at least we know now that

1. Overweight has many *different* causes. Some are found in the world around us, some within the body make-up itself, some stem from emotional pressures, and some are hereditary.
2. Overeating may put the weight on, but it is not a *cause* of overweight.
3. Society shares a major portion of the responsibility for overweight.

But what does this all mean to YOU in terms of licking your individual problem?

No one need tell you about the slings and arrows. You know them only too well, and you react like anyone else to pressure and criticism.

Yet, knowing what to expect, when to expect it, and from *where* to expect it is half the battle.

We've filled you in for good reason. This isn't just another crash diet. It's a three-sided program—remember the diagram on page 6? To get that weight off and keep it off, you need results in all three areas.

But most important of all, you want your good health, good looks, and the good life.

Science is on your side in high gear, so break out your creative imagination, flex those mental muscles, and color you winner!

WHAT'S YOUR OVERWEIGHT RANGE?

The following table gives you a range of heights and weights of teen-agers between the ages of twelve and twenty. The caloric needs listed for each age group are for moderately active teen-agers. Use the table for reference later on when you take your Personal Survey of eating and exercise habits.

If you did not qualify in the Pinch Test, you aren't overfat regardless of how your height and weight show up on the table. Your problem is more mental than physical. You're seeing yourself as fat and judging yourself by unrealistic standards of slimness. So, skip to the ACTION! part and pick out a few exercises to zing you out of the doldrums.

Finding Your Level

Measure your height carefully, without shoes. Then weigh yourself, following the instructions on page 11. Figure that your overweight pounds begin when you are about 15 per cent above average range. Remember that you must allow about ten pounds of growing room before you start thinking about excess weight.

The tables should be used as *guides* only. Girls between eleven and thirteen and boys between twelve and fifteen should be lenient in judging their weight. These are the normal growth-spurt ages when you may gain weight before you gain height.

The final decision as to *exactly* how much excess fat you're carrying is to a great extent arbitrary. Try to be realistic. Your long-range goals may change dramatically if you haven't completed your full growth yet.

How to Weigh Yourself

1. Always weigh yourself once a week at the same time of day, on the same day of the week, and on the same scale.
2. Best time for weighing is in the morning, before breakfast, without clothes. During the day your weight fluctuates by two to four pounds. The morning weight is a better gauge since it remains relatively constant.
3. Check your scale for accuracy and consistency. The scales are important parts of your program (the one in the bathroom and the one you'll be using in the kitchen) and should be the best you can afford.

CHECK FOR ACCURACY: Put something you know the exact weight of (a five-pound bag of flour, for example) on the scale. Any discrepancy must be added to or subtracted from your own weight. (If the scale says the bag of flour weighs seven pounds, you've got to subtract two pounds from your weight each week.)

CHECK FOR CONSISTENCY: Step on the scale, then step off and let it jiggle almost to a stop. Step back on again. Does the needle return to the same weight as before? Does it settle back to zero when you get off it? If not, have the scale repaired or replace it with a new one.

A Couple of Amber Lights

The diets in this book are balanced for the nutritional and caloric needs of the average healthy, but underactive, teen-ager. They are *not* intended for anyone whose diet must be restricted because of specific health problems. The same holds true for the exercises. Check with your doctor first.

For those who are twenty pounds or more overweight, a physical exam and green light from your doctor are *musts*. Get his okay on your Basic Diet Plan and your Exercise Program first; he can help you adjust them to fit your needs.

A complete physical first is a good idea anyway.

HEIGHT-TO-WEIGHT RANGES OF TEEN-AGERS

AGE	SHORT		AVERAGE	
	BOYS	GIRLS	BOYS	GIRLS
12–13	53″–55″ 65–75 lbs.	54″–56″ 65–72 lbs.	58½″–61″ 90–100 lbs.	59″–61″ 92–105 lbs.

Average daily caloric needs: boys, 2,700; girls, 2,300

13–14	55″–57″ 75–80 lbs.	56″–58″ 72–85 lbs.	61″–63½″ 100–115 lbs.	62″–63″ 105–115 lbs.

Average daily caloric needs: boys, 2,700–3,000; girls, 2,300–2,400

14–15	57″–59½″ 80–90 lbs.	58″–60″ 85–90 lbs.	63½″–66″ 115–128 lbs.	63″–63¾″ 115–120 lbs.

Average daily caloric needs: boys, 3,000; girls, 2,400

15–16	59½″–62″ 90–100 lbs.	60″–61″ 90–95 lbs.	66″–67½″ 128–137 lbs.	63¾″–64″ 120–125 lbs.

Average daily caloric needs: boys, 3,000; girls, 2,400, decreasing to 2,300 by age 16

16–17	62″–63″ 100–110 lbs.		67½″–68″ 137–145 lbs.	

Both height and weight gains should taper off for girls during the sixteenth to the seventeenth year. Average height is about 64″; average weight range is between 114 and 126 pounds. After twenty, the daily calorie intake should be reduced to 2,000 for moderately active girls.

TALL		AVERAGE YEARLY GROWTH GAIN	
BOYS	GIRLS	BOYS	GIRLS
64″–67″ *128–145 lbs.*	64″–66″ *125–142 lbs.*	Up to 2½″ *Both: up to 10 lbs.*	Up to 2″
67″–70″ *145–160 lbs.*	66″–67″ *142–150 lbs.*	Up to 3″ *Up to 13 lbs.*	Up to 1½″ *Up to 10 lbs.*
70″–72″ *160–175 lbs.*	67″–68″ *150–160 lbs.*	Up to 2½″ *Up to 13 lbs.*	Up to ¾″ *Up to 6½ lbs.*
72″–73″ *175–185 lbs.*	68″–69″ *160–165 lbs.*	Up to 1½″ *Up to 10 lbs.*	Up to ½″ *Up to 3 lbs.*
73″–73½″ *185–195 lbs.*		Both: up to ¾″ *Both: up to 5½ lbs.*	

Boys usually attain full height by age eighteen. The average height at eighteen is 70″, and average weight is about 150 pounds. Boys' muscular development may continue, and more weight may be added. It may not be extra fat. The Pinch Test will quickly tell if it's fat or muscle. After twenty, boys' daily caloric intake should be reduced to 2,800 for moderately active males.

WHAT'S YOUR HABIT PROFILE?

Let's toss a dash of common sense into the stew. Before you know where you're going, you've got to know where you are. So interview yourself and find out what's happening.

The idea is to analyze your eating and exercise habits and a few of your misconceptions. Be honest and don't kid yourself. Your answers will help you later when you start your program.

Look over the following lists of foods. Check the ones you like:

GROUP 1	GROUP 2	GROUP 3
....Candy (any type)	....Orange	....Green peas
....Rice	....Nuts (any kind)	....Popcorn
....Bread	....Crunchy nibbles	....Cookies
....Potatoes	(crackers, Fritos,	....Strawberries
....Cake	etc.)	....Danish pastries
....Potato chips	....Ice cream sodas/	....Pancakes
....Any vegetables	sundaes/	....Fruits other than
....Mayonnaise/salad	ice milk	orange/
dressing	....Pies	grapefruit/
....Cheese	....Grapefruit	strawberries
....Desserts (all types)	....Butter	
	....Jams/jellies	
	....Sugar	
	....Fried foods	

14

WHAT'S YOUR HABIT PROFILE?

Answer the following:
1. Which of the above foods do you eat every day?
2. Which of the above foods do you dislike?
3. How many regular meals do you eat every day? (A regular meal is a "sit-down" meal with the family at a regular time every day.) ....one ....two ....three ....!....none
4. How many times a day do you eat meat, fish, or poultry? .../.....one ....two ....more ....none
5. How many servings of vegetables do you have each day? ..../....one ....two or more ....none
6. How much bread per day do you eat (include rolls, bagels, crackers, corn bread, biscuits)? ../......very little ....six servings ....more than six
7. Do you eat fried foods at least four times a week? More? *no*
8. How many pieces of fruit do you eat every day? ....one ..../....two or more ....none

How do you rate in activity?
1. What is your favorite leisure-time activity?
2. Which of the following activities do you enjoy and do regularly (i.e., at least four times a week)?

Swimming —	Biking —	Jogging—	Tennis—
Basketball	Volleyball —	Squash	Other..~~Bowling~~
Dancing	Badminton	~~Long walks~~—	

3. How many hours a week are spent in really vigorous exercise? ....X....more than five but less than ten ....between ten and fifteen ....a minimum of fifteen and often more ....none
4. How much time during the day would you estimate that you spend just "hanging around"? ....most of your spare time ....X....half ....almost none

How would you describe your personality?
.........easygoing ....aggressive ....X....quick-tempered
.........anxious ....even-tempered ...X.....tense
....X..ready to take the lead ....don't like being a leader
.........very sociable ...X....don't like to socialize much

With which of the following statements do you agree?

1. Most overweight people lack will power.
2. Eating too much fattening food causes most overweight problems.
3. The best way to lose weight is to take pills to depress the appetite.
4. Losing weight quickly is easiest and is safe.
5. Diet lowers the body's resistance to disease.
6. Skipping meals is a good way to lose weight.
7. Breakfast is the least important meal, so it's usually okay to skip it when you're dieting.
8. Success or failure is all a matter of luck.
9. Like father, like son.
10. What you don't know can't hurt you.
11. Poached eggs are more wholesome than fried eggs.
12. Toast is less fattening than regular bread.
13. Dieters shouldn't drink too much water.

How Do You Score?

We'll give you just a summary. You'll find a lot of the answers as you go along, and some may surprise you. Some of the questions should make you think about your habits.

Come back again after you've read the entire book. Take a look at your answers. Would you answer the questions in the same way the second time?

The three food groups are entirely arbitrary and were done to keep you from unconsciously being dishonest with yourself. If you eat candies, cakes, pies, cookies, potato chips, popcorn, lots of fried foods, ice cream sodas and sundaes, jams, jellies, pastries, crunchy nibbles, you are consuming Cop-out Calories for the most part.

With the exception of ice cream, the foods give you little in return nutritionally. Just calories that add up to pounds.

If you don't eat regular meals (sit-down meals with a full menu) on a regular daily schedule, you are making weight control much more difficult for yourself. A good diet begins with a regular schedule—it's the only way you can start to solve your problem.

A balanced diet gives you at least three servings of meat, poultry, fish, eggs, or cheese every day, three vegetables (in any form—soups, juices, salads), three fruits, breads and cereals, milk, and some fats such as butter and margarine. The dieter eats controlled amounts of all these foods every day.

You are a normally active teen-ager if you get fifteen hours of vigorous exercise every week. If you get more than five but less than ten, you are extremely inactive. If you get *none*, it's time for you to change your program.

If your activity schedule includes plenty of sports, such as those listed previously, and twenty or more hours of vigorous output a week, you are very active and probably in top form. Your main problem is centered in your eating habits and food choices. Keep up the good work. Go to the Basic Diet Plan to help you rearrange your food intake and lower your calories until you lose the excess weight.

Your answers to the personality question should give you a few insights. Researchers have found that the personality pattern of the overweight teen-ager is more passive than that of the normal-weight teen-ager. You are less inclined to actively seek social contacts or to assume leadership roles. And you may not be inclined to stick up for yourself or be healthily aggressive.

If you "see" yourself as easygoing, even-tempered, not wanting to socialize much or to be a leader, you may not be giving yourself an opportunity to really blossom forth!

5

VIVE LA DIFFERENCE!

Owl or Nightingale?

Do you believe Lady Luck smiles on the successful? Is failure due mostly to "bad" luck? If you think so, then you're turning a lovely nightingale into a sour owl.

Thousands of dieters make it in spite of bad luck. Millions of others fail and blame it on luck. Why? What are the essential differences between success and failure?

Basically, there are four simple secrets to success. Again and again, they bubble to the surface of every success story. Put them into *your* program and keep them there, and you've *got to win!* Leave them out, or lose them along the way, and you're asking for trouble.

What are they?

1. You must WANT to succeed

2. You must BELIEVE you can

3. You must give yourself TIME to prove it

4. You must learn to VISUALIZE your goals

Sound simple? It isn't. It's up to you to make the secrets work *for* you. We'll show you how to use them as your basic recipe for success. Add a healthy dash of good nutrition and a pinch of knowledge about what's new from the scientists. Stir in a generous understanding of your emotional needs, and you're ready to brew the stew.

Giving Yourself Time

The first two success secrets are usually present at the beginning of any diet. Once the decision is made, every dieter *wants to succeed* and usually *believes he can.*

Motivation is sky-high at the start. But it drops off rapidly, and zonk goes the diet, back come the pounds.

Any diet program that ignores time will run into a stone wall. *Both mind and body need time to adjust,* and the time varies with each individual.

Many complex changes take place slowly. For instance, some dieters won't lose weight (even on severely restricted diets) for as long as two weeks because their fat cells replace fat loss with water. No actual weight loss shows up until the fat cells "flush" out the water. The dieter who doesn't know this can happen gets disgusted and quits. He's convinced that "anything I eat just turns to fat."

There is mounting evidence to indicate a "trigger" action from fast weight loss. Dropping a lot of pounds quickly apparently can set off a kind of automatic alarm system within the body. The internal mechanisms go into high gear to replace the lost weight. (More about this startling reaction in the next chapter.)

A slow, gradual weight loss seems to get around the problem. It lessens the "shock factor" of too many pounds too fast and gives the body a chance to get accustomed to the changes.

Emotional Backlash

The "shock factor" extends to the realm of the mind, too. Many dieters suffer an emotional backlash from crashing. Some of the backlash comes from not knowing what to expect or how to handle it. Some comes from the internal stresses triggered by a fast weight loss that doesn't give the inner man a period of adjustment.

Fast weight loss can cause severe depression and irritability that may wreck the program. When the pounds return, more guilt and discouragement pile up. In his own mind, and in the minds of others, the dieter shoulders the blame for failure.

Give yourself time to succeed. The period of adjustment is vital to your weight loss program. Without it, you'll never learn to recognize the signals from the inner man that tell you you're right on course.

Remember Your Siamese Triplets

Everyone reacts to the dieter. Expect to make waves. The world around you needs time to adjust to the whole idea, too. Later on, we'll show you some typical reactions and how to handle them.

Visualizing Your Goals

Visualizing your goals unlocks a potent creative force within. It's a technique for flexing the mental muscles, just as you flex your physical muscles.

Visualizing helps you change your self-image as you lose weight. Many teen-agers have virtually starved themselves into the skinnies and continued dieting well past the danger point. Yet they remain firmly convinced that they are still *over-weight!* They still "see" themselves as fat. Nothing can convince them differently because they can't change the *mental* picture they have of themselves.

Getting the Picture

Learn to create a picture in your mind's eye of what you want to achieve. Your total weight loss (thirty pounds, for example) is your long-range goal. This is the mental picture you draw—yourself thirty pounds lighter. Tuck it away firmly and clearly in the back of your mind once you've visualized it completely.

Think of your goal in steps, or intermediate targets. Each five pounds you need to lose should be an intermediate target (in this case, you will have six targets within your overall goal of thirty pounds). Get a clear, mental image of yourself going from the first five-pound target to the second and so on until you reach your long-range goal: a new you in a new way of life.

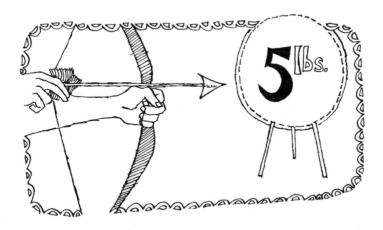

Do not approach your visualizing as if you were simply "thinking" or "daydreaming" about some fanciful ideal. What you're doing is giving the inner man a clear picture of your intentions. You are mentally describing an image that you will actively and positively achieve.

Getting the "Feel" of the Inner Man

The following experiment is a warm-up for the two others that will come later when you're beginning your program. The whole object is to develop a self-awareness and let it grow slowly. Don't rush any of the experiments; give them time to begin working.

EXPERIMENT NO. 1

This experiment will help you develop an eating awareness. Strange as it may seem, this is something most overweights lack. Among overweight teen-agers, pain and tension rather than enjoyment are frequently associated with eating. This isn't surprising since overweights are made to feel "guilty" about eating—regardless of how little or what they eat.

Don't let anything distract your attention while doing the experiment. Try to be alone the first few times you practice it so you can really concentrate on what you're doing.

Be seated at the table with a dish of food before you. Choose one you like from the Basic Proteins Units. Study the food carefully for a few moments, appreciating its color, texture, and aroma. Take a mouthful and chew it slowly, carefully savoring the taste and texture as you chew. Force yourself to eat slowly and to concentrate on an awareness of the food.

Repeat the experiment frequently during the coming weeks. Each time you catch yourself bolting your food, slow down. Quietly and thoroughly chew your food, if only for a few minutes.

If you do the experiment several times a day for two or three weeks, you will become much more alert to poor eating habits and will begin to correct them. You will force yourself to become aware of the kinds of choices you make in foods. This will be your first step toward permanent weight control.

FAT OR FICTION?

FIRST MYTH: The overweight teen-ager is simply overeating.

It ain't necessarily so. Many studies have shown that the great majority of overweight teen-agers *actually consume fewer calories than does the average normal-weight teen-ager.* But they are extremely inactive by comparison! Lack of activity produces the same result as overeating—too many calories taken in, too few expended.

Actually, two distinct groups of overweight teen-agers have been identified by nutrition expert Dr. Mayer. The first group, of course, is the above one. The second group really *does* overeat but exercises normally. Dr. Mayer describes this group as appearing less overfat than the underactive group. Exercise pays dividends in trimmer figures!

In one study, Dr. Mayer and his associates made movies of overweight and normal-weight teen-agers in various types of activities. Analysis of the films revealed that, even in strenuous games, the underactive group was *still underactive.* The actual expenditure of energy by the normal-weight group was *several times* greater than that of the overweights. Most significantly, the overweight teen-agers had no idea that they were less active than their peers.

Born to Be Fat?

In spite of what you may have heard or read to the contrary, heredity does play a part in overweight. Many studies have shown that genetic factors do help to determine whether or not a person will be overfat. This doesn't mean, in a literal sense, that you are "born to be fat." It *does* mean that you may well be *susceptible to overweight*.

For instance, if both your parents are overweight, your chances of following suit are 80%! If one parent is overweight, your chances are 40%. If neither parent is overweight, your chances drop to 10%.

Overweight occurs in certain physical types more frequently than it does in others. Overweight people tend to have heavier, larger bone structures than the average person. And those with long, narrow hands and feet rarely, if ever, become overweight for long. Teen-agers with this type of body build may appear to be fat when they are actually going through a growth spurt. It won't last.

Or Made to Be Fat?

It is quite true that family eating patterns can set the stage for weight problems. Many parents still cling to the belief that a fat baby is a healthy baby. The overeating/underactivity pattern begins with overfeeding the baby.

By the time the child reaches seven or eight, the habits have become a "norm." Overeating is mistakenly encouraged; for example, the child is prompted to finish the food on his plate or have second and third helpings when he really isn't hungry. Frequently, the family diet may be too high in fats and carbohydrates such as breads, cakes, heavy gravies, rice, pasta, and food cooked with too much fat.

Some overeating is due to ignorance of what an average portion of food really is. Many children are brought up on food portions several times the size actually needed for caloric balance. Three or four pork chops, for instance, may be just right for a Green Bay Packer, but they are two more than the average person needs.

Appetite or Hunger?

Many people lump appetite and hunger together. But the two *are* different, and the difference may be of special importance to the dieter.

Appetite is essentially a pleasant sensation of desire for, or anticipation of, food one enjoys. It involves the senses of smell, taste, and sight.

Research shows that the overweight are far more sensitive to these external stimulations than normal-weight persons. Such sensitivity explains in part why some overweights will eat when they couldn't possibly be *hungry* or physically in need of food.

Hunger is usually an unpleasant sensation. How unpleasant depends upon how long one has gone without food. Some of its symptoms are: stomach pangs, nausea, dizziness, headaches, tiredness. Reactions vary widely among individuals.

Regulation of Food Intake

Scientists have found that the appetite is controlled by a satiety (or fullness) center called the "appestat." It is a small section of the hypothalamus gland located in the brain. Right beside the appestat is the "feeding center" that stimulates man to eat. Apparently, the feeding center is constantly active and the appestat acts as a brake to stop feeding after a certain point is reached.

What triggers the appestat, and when, is still a mystery. A number of little-understood chemical and biological reactions may stimulate the appestat to put on the brakes. Some experts suspect that unknown hormones may be the answer.

Overweights tend to be much less sensitive than normal-weights to the internal signals of satiety. Thus, overeaters will continue to eat beyond the normal cut-off point—until they "feel" full. Sadly enough, the full feeling is *not necessarily a feeling of satiety* but often is a muscular discomfort resulting from having stuffed the stomach to the limits of its capacity.

More Startling Clues!

Dr. Walter Bortz, of Lankenau Hospital in Philadelphia, has found that there is a metabolic similarity between the well-fed fat person and a starving lean person. (*Metabolism* is the scientific word to describe the rate at which the body burns food.)

Dr. Bortz discovered that the well-fed fat person was chemically burning up more fat (called high fat utilization) and relatively less blood sugar than is normal. This "metabolic setting" is the same for a starving lean person.

When the lean person faces acute starvation, his system goes into high gear, enabling him to reach a peak level of fat utilization. Dr. Bortz found that this peak level *was already in effect in the fat person!*

But, obviously, the well-fed fat person isn't starving, and has no need for such a metabolic setting. So what is happening?

In effect, the fat person is *hibernating*. It's really a hangover from ancient times when people survived periods of little or no food by living on their storage of body fat. Many wild animals still do this. During periods of plenty, their bodies anticipate future needs by storing up fat for later use.

Dr. Bortz's research may give us important clues as to why so many dieters regain their lost weight. The body may seek to reset itself at a weight level far higher than is needed in today's world. Such a reaction suggests the possibility that some people could be *genetically programmed* to start the hibernation cycle in anticipation of future needs.

Or the hibernation cycle could be triggered by false feast-or-famine clues from crash dieting. Crash diets are calorically restricted diets that put an enormous pressure on the body in a short time span. In effect, they are intense periods of starvation that may be compared to yelling "FIRE!" in a crowded auditorium. They push the panic button and send the whole complex system into high gear. The more frequently one crash diets, the more frequently he reinforces the feast-or-famine response.

So chalk up a good, strong reason for the third success secret: TIME. The more gradual your weight loss, the better chance you have of avoiding the "rebound effect"—gaining back the lost pounds with added interest.

FOOD OR FODDER?

Most dieters are impatient for results and want miracles overnight. They jump at any scheme that promises to deliver. Unfortunately, many highly touted fad diets are nutritional copouts. Sure, they work—at your expense.

The overweight teen-ager is a very different breed of cat from the overweight adult. Good nutrition is basic to good health at any age, but for the teen-ager, it is absolutely essential. You're in the last great growth cycle, and you need certain basic foods every day, just for growing.

But a diet doesn't have to be dull or short-circuit your health. In fact, there is some evidence that a low-calorie diet lacking rich nutritional variety will actually defeat your purpose. It seems that weight is more easily controlled in teenagers with diets high in nutritional values, even if they are slightly higher in calories!

Yet, there are simple tricks for cutting calories without sacrificing good eating, taste, or fun.

The Basic Six: What You Need to Grow On

Scientists have identified over fifty different elements, or chemical substances, in food. These substances are grouped into six major classes called "nutrients."

The Basic Six are proteins, carbohydrates, vitamins, minerals, fats, and water. One other element—not strictly a nutrient but highly important in the nutritional chain—is air.

The real bulk of all foods are proteins, carbohydrates,

28

fats, and water. Many of the minerals and vitamins are only needed in minute amounts, but scientists agree that *all* are necessary in a balanced diet.

Only three of the Basic Six contain calories: the proteins, carbohydrates, and fat. Calories are units of measurement, as are inches or quarts. When the body "burns" food, it releases energy in the form of heat that can be measured. One unit of energy (one calorie) is equal to the heat needed to raise the temperature of two quarts of water 1°F.

> **SECOND MYTH:** *People gain weight because they eat too much fattening food.*

Do they? Proteins and carbohydrates contain four calories per gram. Fat has nine. The difference is in the *concentration* of calories. Proteins and carbohydrates contain more water, and fiber, ounce for ounce, than fat does. But *all calories are alike*. Four protein calories are precisely equal to four fat calories. So there is really no such thing as a "fattening" food!

For instance, butter (a fat) and honey (a carbohydrate) are both highly concentrated—the calories are packed into a small space. But an orange is about 88% water, so the calories are scattered around. It takes over four pounds of oranges to equal the calories in 3½ ounces of butter. Yet, as far as the body is concerned, the calories (about 716) are identical from either source.

The *nutritional* difference between the two is another story. The amounts and proportions of the Basic Six in butter are quite different from those in oranges. This is true among all foods, and *this is the reason for planning a diet!* One food, or one limited group of foods, can't give you all the nutrients you need to grow on.

The Missing Ingredient

Until recently, recognition of one major ingredient in nutrition was missing: TIME.

Long-term effects of nutrition are difficult to measure. The human being is an unsatisfactory guinea pig. He takes too long to grow, mature, and reproduce more generations of offspring for study. This has been one of the big stumbling blocks in pinpointing causes of obesity and in distinguishing between genetic and nutritional causes.

But luckily for us—and especially for teen-agers—scientists have proven two very important nutritional points:

First, they have proven that certain nutrients are *essential* for growth, health, and maintenance of life. We now know what the nutrients are and how much we need every day. We also know that other nutrients, called "trace elements" because they are so minute, are equally essential.

Second, the scientists have proven that the growing years are nutritionally the most important. They are the building years when a good balance of essential nutrients pays off in good health dividends for life.

You've probably heard that "you are what you eat." For the teen-ager, it should be said, "YOU WILL BE WHAT YOU EAT."

Brass Tacks

There are hundreds of "sure-fire" diets that rely on a few restricted foods guaranteed to shave pounds. The quacks assure you these diets are balanced so you don't need variety.

The reason for variety is sound and simple: all nutrients interact with each other. Each one gives a helping hand to the other in the body's chemistry. Nutritionists urge variety in diet so that you can be sure you're getting the essential interaction.

For example, for the body to use niacin, an important B vitamin, it needs help from an amino acid found in whole protein. So you couldn't say, "Ah! Poppycock Biscuits give me my minimum daily requirement of niacin, so I'll eat one every day to be sure." Without help from protein, which may not be in Poppycock Biscuits, your body would be unable to use the niacin. *The same principle holds true in dozens of other cases.*

The nutritionists are simply saying that variety is the spice of life. There are no miracle foods, no miracle diets. You can lose weight on any food, even ice cream. And you can lose a lot of weight quickly. But to lose it safely and healthfully, your first concern should be with good nutrition.

REV IT UP!

Double-talk nonsense. The calories you consume have an unchanging relationship to the energy you use up.

All foods contain calories. Your body burns them every minute, awake or asleep. The more active you are, the more calories you burn simply because you are expending more energy.

The equation is this: 3,500 calories equal one pound of body fat. If you don't use the 3,500 calories in energy output, your body socks them away in the fat bank.

The relationship between caloric input (eating and drinking) and energy output (exercise and just the process of living) is called "caloric balance."

Normal-weight people are in caloric balance because their output equals their input. Their daily caloric intake may vary widely, but *over a span of time,* their bodies will automatically readjust the input-output balance. In effect, their appestats put the brakes on until their activity levels rise.

The overweights can't rely on this automatic process. They must *deliberately* set about adjusting the balance.

The only known way a healthy person can lose weight is by consuming fewer calories than he expends in energy. But hold on!

Most people think that means, "I've got to cut calories." Not necessarily so! You can readjust your caloric balance by keeping your caloric intake at its normal level but *increasing your energy output.* The net effect is still an input-output gap.

For the overweight teen-ager who is *underactive* but who is not *overeating,* this is the most sensible approach. Your Habit Profile Test on page 14 should give you a clue as to your category. If you still can't decide, make your decision after you've taken the Personal Survey for one week.

It makes no difference if the calories are going in or going out; they MUST BE ACCOUNTED FOR EITHER WAY. Put that up in neon lights! You can bet your beads that any diet that gets results means someone has counted the calories in both directions. You can't lose weight without an input/output gap.

> *FOURTH MYTH: Exercise is of no value in losing weight.*

Let's bury this one once and for all. The "calorie-cutting school" cites horrifying examples of how much strenuous exercise you need in order to use up 3,500 calories (thus one pound). Many a poor dieter has said, quite rightly, "I could lose weight if I got more exercise." But he has a nightmare vision of killing himself with "dangerous" exercise before he can get results. Ergo, exercise is of little value.

Lumping all your exercise together is like trying to get your fifty-six hours of weekly sleep in one stretch. If you divide exercise into segments, just as you do sleep, you still get the same benefits. It makes no difference whether you use up 3,500 calories in one lump or a dozen segments. The result is one pound less either way.

But—when you pace your exercise program in the same way you pace your diet program—*you get added dividends.* The ACTION! chapter tells you all about it.

There's one more clincher the buffoons of the bulges use to put down exercise:

FIFTH MYTH: *Exercise increases the appetite, so you eat more and gain back the weight.*

Scientists have found that a moderate amount of regular exercise helps to control the appetite. Sedentary living actually increases it!

Even heavy, vigorous exercise puts you ahead of the game. For instance, if you spent the day skiing (*really* skiing, not standing around watching), you could use up at least 6,000 calories. Even if you came back with a monstrous appetite and gulped down 5,000 calories—no mean task—you would still have a calorie deficit. Inevitably, you would *not* eat as many calories as you had spent in energy.

In a nutshell: exercise helps to control the appetite and maintain the gap between input and output.

Yep, that's the way it works, and it's been proven.

EATING TO LIVE

Proteins

The first essential for good health is protein, the master builder, so-called because it is basic to all living cells.

Your growing years are peak demand periods for protein. But protein needs continue throughout life. The body needs protein to build new bone and muscle tissues as you grow. In addition, the body uses protein to repair and maintain cells and to replace the millions of cells that die every day.

There's no substitute for it. It can't be stored, and the body can't manufacture it from other nutrients. If you don't eat enough protein to meet your daily needs, your body will raid its own muscle tissues to get the needed protein.

Protein is made up of substances called amino acids, a number of which are essential. (Classifying a nutrient as "essential" means the body must get it from the foods you eat—the body can't make up its own.)

Whole or complete proteins contain all the essential amino acids. Incomplete proteins lack one or more.

All animal foods, except gelatin, are complete protein foods. This includes animal products such as eggs, milk, and cheese.

Plants are important but secondary sources of protein. In comparison with animal foods, they furnish protein in much smaller amounts. Most plant proteins are incomplete. The best and most efficient plant proteins come from soybeans and other dried legumes.

Best sources of proteins are: animal foods—veal, liver, beef, pork, lamb, turkey, chicken, eggs, fish, milk, cheese;

plant foods—soybeans, dried beans and peas, nuts, whole-grain cereals and breads.

Minerals

1592826

Minerals are vital keystones to body metabolism. Without them, the other nutrients can't do their work.

For the teen-ager, iron and calcium are the minerals most likely to be deficient in the diet. Iron is a blood builder and is essential in the transport of oxygen to the body cells. Calcium is important in building strong bones and teeth and in regulating the heartbeat.

The best sources of these two minerals are the whole-protein foods—meat, poultry, fish, milk, cheese—together with the dark leafy green vegetables, dried beans and peas.

Fortunately, by taking care of your protein, iron, and calcium needs, you will usually provide enough of the other minerals needed by the body (phosphorus, potassium, copper, sodium, for example).

Vitamins

These constitute the "newest" group of nutrients. Identifying them has been extremely difficult because of the small quantities involved. But vitamins are all out of proportion in importance!

Vitamins have been called the "coordinators" because they work with each other and with other nutrients in building and maintaining health.

Scientists have discovered thirteen vitamins—all essential to good health. Recommended daily allowances have been established for all but two: K and D.

Six vitamins are considered major nutrients in planning a balanced diet. Variety in the diet will usually supply the minute quantities needed of the other seven.

VITAMIN A: helps growth and repair of body tissues; is necessary for good vision, soft, smooth skin, and healthy mucous membranes.
Best sources: liver, carrots, sweet potatoes, squash, cantaloupe, dark green leafy vegetables.

THIAMINE (B₁): is essential in heart, nerve, and muscle functioning, in converting carbohydrates to energy, and in digestion and assimilation of foods.

Best sources: pork, dried beans and peas, liver, lamb, veal, nuts, whole-grain cereals.

RIBOFLAVIN (B₂): helps maintain good vision; helps cells use oxygen; is necessary for good skin and mouth tissues and for vitality and efficiency.

Best sources: liver, poultry, beef, veal, lamb, pork, oysters, fish, cottage cheese, flour and cereal products. Liver once a week plus regular use of leafy green vegetables and milk assures a high level of intake.

NIACIN (a B VITAMIN): like thiamine and riboflavin, niacin is concerned with helping cells to use oxygen. It aids in smooth functioning of the nervous system and is necessary for maintaining a healthy skin and tongue.

Best sources: meat, poultry, fish, flour and cereal products.

VITAMIN C (ASCORBIC ACID): its most important function is forming and maintaining a substance that binds living cells together, helping body fluids to nourish them. It builds resistance to infection, hastens healing, is necessary in utilization of iron, and helps build and maintain bones, tissues, and blood.

Best sources: oranges, grapefruits, strawberries, lemons, cantaloupes, tomatoes, broccoli, dark green leafy vegetables, and tropical fruits such as papayas, which are often available in supermarkets.

VITAMIN D: is important in promoting normal growth; combines with calcium and phosphorus to build bones and teeth.

Best sources: fish liver oil, liver, fortified milk, and eggs.

Note: Since ultraviolet rays are a major source of Vitamin D, it is called the "sunshine" vitamin. It is added to milk in order to insure adequate amounts of that vitamin in the average diet throughout the year.

Carbohydrates

These are sugars and starches, and they are found in most foods. The word "carbohydrates" is used as a blanket term to describe classes of foods that are composed mainly of starch or of sugar. Typical ones are: breads, cereals, sweets of all types, pastas, syrups, table sugars.

Carbohydrates provide energy. They are important in carrying on the work of the muscles and the internal body processes. Cellulose, a starchlike substance found in bulky vegetables (celery, for example), plays an important role in the digestive processes.

Excess carbohydrates can be converted into fat and used as such. Or they can be stored as fat in the fat cells.

Fats

The main sources of fats are butter, margarine, salad oils, meat fats, nuts, cheese, cream, whole milk.

Fats provide energy, a feeling of satiety, or fullness, and are bearers of vitamins. Fat deposits within the body also cushion and protect vital organs and help in heat retention.

Many health professionals think the American diet is too high in fats and they urge cutting down. Since fats are highly concentrated sources of calories, cutting fat consumption is necessary for weight control.

However, since proteins and carbohydrates can be converted into fat, *all* foods are a potential source of body fat. Stored body fat (as in overweight) reflects the total amount of *all foods* eaten in excess of energy needs.

Water and Air

Though neither is a food, they are nevertheless recognized as essential nutrients.

Water is the major solvent for all nutrients. It transports nutrients and waste materials, acts as a cushion to protect vital organs, aids in regulation of body temperature, acts as a lubricant at the joints, and is essential in building and repairing body tissues.

Air provides oxygen for the all-important combustion process—the burning of the body's fuel, food.

The following chart shows which foods are the best sources of the various nutrients.

Proteins→ beef · veal · lamb · pork · turkey · chicken · eggs · fish · milk · cheeses · soybeans · gelatin · dried beans, peas · nuts · whole grain cereals, bread · peanut butter · dark green leafy vegetables·

Minerals: calcium→ milk · cheese · sardines · dark green leafy vegetables · fish · eggs · broccoli · sweet potato · cabbage · orange - grapefruit · dried fruit · canteloup · molasses · bread·

iron→ liver · all meats · oysters · fish · poultry · eggs · dried beans, peas · dark green leafy vegetables · molasses, nuts, dried fruits

Carbohydrates→ ♡ · sugars - syrups · molasses · cereals · breads · flour and flour products · potatoes · honey · jellies · jams · candies and other sweets · starchy vegetables·

Vitamins — dried fruits · eggs · cheese ·
liver · sweet potato · carrots ·
spinach · canteloup · asparagus ·
winter squash · dark
green leafy vegetables ·
tomatoes · broccoli ·

A

B — Thiamine: pork · dried beans
and peas · liver · lamb · veal ·
nuts · peas · potato · orange ·
oysters · poultry · fish ·
Riboflavin: liver · all meats ·
oysters · fish · cottage cheese ·
milk · cheese · spinach · squash ·
asparagus · bread · cereals ·
Niacin: all meats, especially
organ meats · tuna fish · poultry ·
fish · peanut butter · dried fruits ·
potato · peas · dried beans and
peas, breads and cereals ·

C — orange · grapefruits · strawberries · canteloup · lemons ·
tomatoes · broccoli · dark green
leafy vegetables · cabbage · potato ·
green pepper · asparagus · peas ·
lettuce · liver · papayas · guava ·
mango · tangerine · green beans ·
cauliflower · okra ·

D — liver · fish liver oil · eggs ·
fortified milk ·

FATS: Butter · lard · salad oils, dressings ·
margarine · meat and poultry
fats · bacon · nuts · mayonnaise ·
creams · vegetable shortening ·
gravies · many cheeses ·

10

ON YOUR MARK

If you want to grow up slim and stay that way there are only two things you must do:

You must **EXERCISE**.

You must **EAT**.

Eating means breakfast, lunch, dinner, and at least two snacks—one at mid-morning (whenever possible) and the other in mid-afternoon. No skipping meals or letting yourself get overhungry, and no calorie shortchanging. Your minimum daily intake should equal 1,800 calories for girls, 2,200 for boys.

It's really common sense. Your long-range goal is to get the weight off and keep it off. You've got to learn new eating habits and new exercise habits. Starvation dieting doesn't retrain the inner man. Nor will you get the pounds off while warming the bench.

Start your weight control by setting up a regular eating schedule and a regular exercise schedule. Skipping meals, grabbing nutritionally empty snacks, foraging for what's left in the refrigerator—all throw your regulating machinery out of whack. Sticking to a regular eating schedule balances your body processes and makes weight control a lot easier.

So don't try to cop out with the standard teen-ager's excuse, "I don't have the time!" If you really want to get those pounds off, you'll find it. You must be as stubborn as a mule about your diet/exercise schedule and as tenacious as a bull-dog.

Rearrange your out-of-school schedule around diet and exercise and let other things fall into place. You'll find it's basically a more natural rhythm anyway. All of those passive activities that cost time and pounds will balance out in better proportion. The results will be a healthier and happier life.

Why Eat?

Man is by nature a nibbling animal, and frequent feedings are his natural pattern. The routine three meals a day are convenient accommodations to work and social schedules, not to appetite.

Doctors working with the overweight have found that frequent feedings (about six a day) are helpful in controlling appetite and regulating the body's metabolism. Dr. Frederick Stare, of Harvard, calls this "scientific nibbling," and he has recommended it to his dieters for many years.

But the "scientific nibble" is quite different from the usual nibble. You divide your total food allowance into smaller portions and eat more frequently. The mid-morning, mid-afternoon, or late-evening nibble, then, should be part of the food you would normally eat at a regular meal.

The Basic Diet Plan provides for three between-meal nibbles a day. Some of you will find it difficult, or impossible, to eat your mid-morning snack because of your school schedule. In such cases, add the food to breakfast or lunch.

The mid-morning snack is important in helping to curb the appetite. If nothing interferes with your having a snack at that time, don't neglect it! In any event, do not eliminate the food just because you can't manage to eat it during mid morn ing.

If you're under the illusion that you cut calories by skipping breakfast (or any meal), forget it! You more than make up for it later when the hunger whammies hit and you're ready to eat anything that isn't nailed down.

Breakfast is more than your energy meal to begin the day. It's your first appetite-control meal. Don't skip it. A balanced energy breakfast (with a protein) raises your blood sugar level, which helps ward off both excessive hunger and the mid-morning lows.

What's in a Portion?

Knowing portions accurately is your first step to calorie control. You must have a very clear, *visual* idea of just how big or how little any given amount of food is. Do you know what a three-ounce hamburger looks like? How much space in your juice glass does four ounces of orange juice occupy?

You will need three things when you begin your diet: a small postal scale, a measuring cup, and a measuring spoon. You will need to weigh or measure most food portions at least once in order to become familiar with them. Correct measurements are crucial with concentrated-calorie foods such as fats and some carbohydrates.

Measures

Don't confuse measurements by weight with measurements by volume. They are two different things entirely, even though they may occasionally coincide. For instance, three quarters of a cup of puffed wheat does *not* equal six ounces. The "six ounces" marked on the side of the cup refers to liquid, or volume, measurements only. (See the endpapers of this book for tables giving common measurements by weight and measurements by volume.)

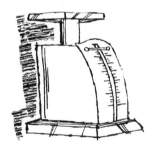

More and more manufacturers are putting calorie counts of foods on the package label. Usually it's a sincere attempt to be helpful. But it can be used to deliberately mislead, particularly on some so-called "low-calorie" foods. Just be on your toes and make comparisons with the regular product. Be sure you use a common measure for both.

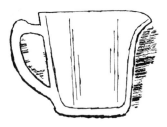

In general, low-calorie foods should be used with caution. Many products relied on cyclamates (which have now been banned) and on saccharin (now under suspicion as a possible cause of cancer) to lower the calories. Until the scientists come up with a truly safe additive that cuts the calories, the dieter's best friend is a re-education of eating habits firmly married to an active, busy life.

(Incidentally, the label "low-calorie" isn't license to gorge! Most foods have enough calories to add up if you eat too much. Some may be only one or two calories lower than the regular product.)

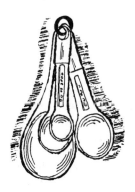

11

OKAY, ALFIE,
WHAT'S IT ALL ABOUT?

Mostly, it's about eating for good health while you erase those excess pounds. But let's be candid.

When you first start a diet, it's extra work. You'll stop to think about what goes on the shopping list. In the grocery store, you'll change some "grab" habits for some stop and choose ones. In the kitchen, you will pause to count calories and portions for judicious cutting. Occasionally, you'll go out of your way to put more eyeball appeal into your menu.

But you will teach yourself many important things about eating for good and lasting health. Once they're down pat, the good food habits will be no more trouble than the bad food habits.

Calorie control and good nutrition both begin with food choice and correct portions. Keep your menus simple at first until you get accustomed to correct portions and new patterns of food selection.

The common sense of weight control is simply cutting down or eliminating high-calorie foods and substituting other foods. It may not mean a lesser amount of food. In fact, for many dieters, it may actually mean *more* food!

Your Diet Needs

Teen-agers need a slightly different diet from adults. If you follow the basic plan in choosing foods, you will get a high-quality diet with a minimum calorie cost—the best food for the price.

The emphasis on leafy green vegetables, vegetable juices, and soups provides for your iron and Vitamin A needs (in addition to other great plus factors). The diet offers dividends for those with skin problems. Strict control of fats, coupled with lots of vegetables and fruits, helps give you a healthy, glowing skin. (More on skin care later.)

If you like liver and other organ meats, plan a serving once a week. These meats are especially rich in iron and the B vitamins. But most American teen-agers simply won't eat organ meats. A good supply of top-quality, iron-rich vegetables will solve the problem.

Part of the anti-liver sentiment stems from the habit of overcooking it. Try the recipe on page 86 for a method of cooking that makes liver a delicious treat instead of a tough, gray shingle. Don't forget that chicken livers count as a liver serving, too!

The Basic Diet Plan is high in proteins and allows many choices. In general, your daily eating pattern should include one protein choice from eggs, cheese, or dried peas/beans. The other two choices should come from meat, poultry, or fish. If you enjoy seafood, have it often. Boys have one extra Protein Unit and two extra Breads/Cereals Units that should be added in each day.

The fat allowance in the Basic Diet Plan depends upon your selecting (and eating) lean meats trimmed of *all visible* fat. It also depends upon keeping your eyes open for hidden calories in frying, sautéing, in sauces, gravies, and salad mixes.

Watch Your Calories

Think of all butter, margarine, oils, and fats as foods with calories. When you add them to other foods, the *total* calories must be counted. For example, if you scramble an egg in a Teflon pan (which requires no fat to prevent food from sticking to the pan), you have only 77 calories. But scramble the same egg in one tablespoon of margarine and you get 177 calories!

Keep a sharp eye on your breads and cereals, too. They can make your calorie intake skyrocket if you get careless.

The fact that vegetables aren't figured in your caloric intake doesn't mean that calories don't count. But vegetables are so low in calories and so high in bulk that they aren't likely to blow your diet—*if* you follow the Basic Diet Plan.

The few vegetables that are portion-controlled are italicized on the list of vegetables. All vegetables should be cooked without butter, fats, and sauces, unless you use your Fats Unit (or Breads/Cereals—if it's flour) from your daily allowance.

Your high intake of vegetables and vegetable juices acts as a low-calorie appetite control. The calorie counts on the lists of Food Units are for your use in figuring total calories in dishes you may want to make from recipes.

How's It Done?

The Basic Diet Plan is set up in Units, precalculated to give you correct calorie and nutrition control. If you lose weight too rapidly, you *must* add back into your daily diet more Food Units until your rate of weight loss has adjusted to the correct level.

If you aren't losing fast enough, a quick glance at your daily menu sheets will tell if you've added too much food. But if you're following the minimum allowance as shown, then you know your EXERCISE UNITS are too low. *Never deduct food below your minimum allowances.*

The Basic Diet Plan gives you nutritional protection while letting you spot exactly where your problems are in your weight control program.

The Calorie Charts in the back of the book give you added counts in common ingredients used in standard recipes. Use it to figure calories in an average serving.

Use the Basic Diet Units with the Calorie Chart to figure your Diet Units in any recipe. Stew, for example, might have one Protein Unit, two Fats Units, one Breads/Cereals Unit and a Vegetable Unit.

Your Menus

Plan your menus by the week. This will let you get lots of variety in foods (you can see the whole week at a glance), and you or your family can make the most of your food money. Leftovers can be planned for and used in other dishes.

A serving of meat is about three ounces of *cooked edible* lean portion. It does not include bone or fat. Until you reach your proper weight level, all foods should be broiled, roasted, boiled, baked, or steamed.

Some fried foods are listed. Don't use them more than once a week. The protein sacrifice is too great since you must reduce the portion to make up for extra calories gained in frying.

Fried breaded foods are really off limits until you're well into your maintenance program and can increase your calorie intake to normal levels.

Calorie allowances for meats are based on standard lean cuts as found in most supermarkets. If you don't trim cuts and select for leanness, you add back hundreds of calories every month. Prime cuts are MUCH higher in calories (sometimes almost double!) since they are liberally marbled with fat.

Pork is perfectly acceptable and an excellent source of valuable nutrients. Choose for minimum fat such lean cuts as loin, center cut ham, and carefully trim out excess fat from any pork. You can cut many calories from pork, especially bacon and sausage, by cooking crisply and draining well.

The dieter frequently comes out better nutritionally by choosing pork over other protein foods. Five slices of crisply fried, well-drained Canadian bacon have a lot more nutritional zap than, say, two franks—at the same calorie cost!

Broil and roast all meats on racks so the fats can drain off. Use Teflon pans for frying and scrambling eggs and for nonfatty meats.

Any butter, margarine, fats, or oil used in cooking must be counted as one or more of your Basic Fats Units.

Cook vegetables quickly in as little water as possible to avoid losing valuable vitamins and minerals. Overcooking destroys vitamins, and too much water washes them away.

Save the juices in which you have cooked vegetables. They are loaded with good nutrition. Store them in the refrigerator. Try mixing your own combinations for quick pickups.

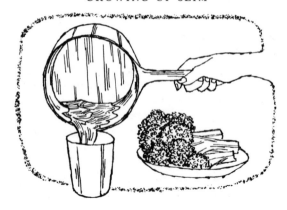

A cold glass of fresh vegetable juice just before lunch or dinner can do wonders to curb a pesky appetite.

Keep a supply of small, six-ounce cans of V-8 juice in the refrigerator as part of your emergency supplies. Calorie costs are negligible—less than thirty a can—vitamin and mineral content is high.

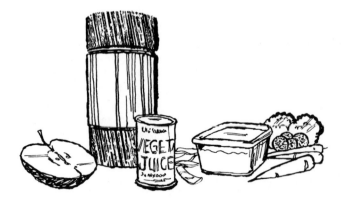

Substitute a piece of lean, nonfat pork for ham or bacon if you like a touch of meat flavor in cooked leafy vegetables.

12

ABOUT THE BASIC DIET PLAN

You need not stick to a set pattern of food distribution throughout the day, except for one or two things.

First, breakfast should include a protein—either a complete Unit or a part of one.

Second, your food intake should be spread out across the day. This simply means don't drink your whole quart of milk for breakfast or eat all of your protein at dinner!

The Basic Diet Plan lists "maximum calories" in several places. That's for beginning dieters who must watch their calories closely. For instance, girls on 1,800 calories a day must choose a *minimum* of three Protein Units but must not exceed their *maximum* daily calorie allowance of 750 from the Basic Proteins list.

You are allowed up to 250 calories for each Protein Unit. Some of them are less, particularly the fish. So you may have calories left over for choosing another fruit or protein (without exceeding your allowance).

If you choose three beef proteins in one day, however, you might not have any elbowroom, and you could overshoot your mark. That's why variety is your keynote: it averages everything out.

Divide your food in any way you want. For instance, you may eat one quarter of a cantaloupe at breakfast and save the other quarter for mid-afternoon. Or you may have one egg for breakfast and the other at dinner in a vegetable dish.

Your three snacks a day should emphasize vegetables and vegetable juices and fruits. Eat as many fresh vegetables as you like. Keep plenty on hand at all times. Page 81 gives you a recipe for a High-Protein Vegetable Dip.

Later in your program, you will need to increase your food intake as you increase your activity level in order to keep your weight loss at the correct average. But don't increase Cop-out Calories! Instead, select from the Basic Units in this order: proteins, milk, fruits, fats, breads/cereals. Vegetables can be increased any time.

YOUR BASIC DIET PLAN

Daily Calorie Allowance: **Basic Units of**		*Girls 1,800*	*Boys 2,200*
Protein	*Minimum Choices:	3 units	4 units
	Maximum:	*750 calories*	*1,000 calories*
Milk	*Minimum Choices:	4 units	4½ units
	Maximum:	*348 calories*	*390 calories*
Fats	Choices:	3 units	3 units
	Maximum:	*155 calories*	*155 calories*
Breads/ Cereals	Choices:	6 units	8 units
	Maximum:	*360 calories*	*480 calories*
Fruits	*Minimum Choices:	3 units	3 units
	Maximum:	*175 calories*	*175 calories*
Vegetables	Minimum Choices:	3 units	3 units
Soup	Minimum Choices:	5 a week	5 a week

* If you have extra calories left over, you may add one of these Units to your menu, as long as you don't exceed your daily calorie *total.*

ABOUT THE BASIC DIET PLAN

BASIC PROTEIN UNITS
Any portion listed is a Unit

Boys: 4 a day, minimum
Maximum calories: 1,000 from the Basic Protein Units for your Basic Diet Plan of 2,200 calories

Girls: 3 a day, minimum
Maximum calories: 750 from the Basic Protein Units for the Basic Diet Plan of 1,800 calories

All portions are cooked portions and include ONLY the lean edible part. You will need to weigh most protein foods, as cooked, when you first begin so you can learn to judge by eye. In general, three cooked ounces is about four ounces raw, trimmed.

	Average Calories
Beef	
3 ounces, any lean cut with all visible fat removed: eye round, top or bottom round, lean, ground round (for hamburger/meat loaf), flank steak, sirloin, stew meat (six 1″ cubes), pot roast, rump, tenderloin, rib of beef, organ meats (such as brains, liver, kidneys), tongue (4 slices about 3 x 2 x ⅛)	245

	Average Calories
Veal	
3 ounces, any lean veal: cutlet, roast, stew meat, chop	195
Pork	
3 ounces, any lean portion: chop, ham, loin, liver, tenderloin. Ham may be smoked, cured, cooked, or fresh.	240
5 slices Canadian bacon, crisp, drained	250
2 links sausage (3 x ½) or 1 sausage patty, cooked well, drained (2 oz. when raw)	250

Lamb	Average Calories	Fish (cont'd)	Average Calories
3 ounces, any lean portion: chop, roast leg or breast, lamb burgers (ground from lean cut without added fat)	258	catfish, cod, flounder, haddock, halibut, mackerel, trout	192
		1 broiled lobster (1½ pounds)	216

Chicken

3 ounces, any lean portion: roasted, baked, stewed — 256

½ breast, Southern fried (see recipes), or — 232

2 medium legs, or
1 leg, 1 thigh, or
1 small breast, baked, roasted, stewed, or
¼ small broiler — 200

Turkey

3 ounces, any lean portion (including pressed turkey or turkey roll) — 228

Fish (All baked or broiled; no Fats Units included)

4 ounces any fresh or frozen fish: bass, bluefish, carp,

(To round out a fish dinner, you may want clams on the half shell or shrimp; see the listings for other foods in the index.)

¾ cup water- or oil-packed tuna fish, *drained* — 240

¾ cup salmon, including bones, skin — 168

1 can sardines, drained (3¾ oz. size) — 190

Eggs, Cheese, Legumes

2 eggs, cooked, without butter — 154

4 slices American cheese — 210

2 ounces cheddar, other hard cheese — 230

¾ cup cottage cheese — 162

¾ cup cooked dried beans/peas — 230

ABOUT THE BASIC DIET PLAN

BASIC MILK UNITS
Portion listed is a Unit

GIRLS: 4 cups a day, minimum   BOYS: 4½ cups a day, minimum
   Maximum calories: 348   Maximum calories: 390

1 cup of nonfat skimmed milk or nonfat buttermilk, 86 calories. You may use the milk with cereal, in soups, in dishes you cook. But *you must use the daily minimum.*
Whole milk has twice the number of calories, so you cannot add it to your diet until you have reached your weight goal and are well into maintenance—and remaining vigorously active.
Note: The powdered nonfat skimmed milk (fortified) is lowest in calories (86/87 a cup) and is recommended. Mix it several hours before use and let it chill thoroughly for best flavor.

BASIC FATS UNITS
Any portion listed is a Unit
Minimum daily allowance: 3
Maximum calorie allowance for Basic Diet Plan: 155

	Average Calories		Average Calories
1 teaspoon of butter or margarine	35	1 teaspoon shortening	37
1 slice bacon, crisp, well-drained	50	1 teaspoon bacon fat	42
2 tablespoons light cream (sweet, sour)	60	1 teaspoon chicken fat	42
1 tablespoon heavy cream	50	1 teaspoon lard (pure)	42
1 heaping tablespoon whipped cream	50	1 teaspoon olive oil	41
1 tablespoon cream cheese	55	2 teaspoons peanut butter	60
1 tablespoon French dressing	70	6 small nuts (pecan, filbert, walnut, almond, peanut, etc.)	45
1 teaspoon mayonnaise	35	2 brazil nuts	56
1 teaspoon salad dressing	35	1 tablespoon coconut, shredded	42
1 tablespoon gravy	80	6 small olives, plain, green or black	40
1 teaspoon vegetable oil	42	3 large olives, plain, green or black	36

Note that bacon can be used as a Fats Unit and is included in the list. Use the Unit in recipes but do not count it in with a Protein Unit. Keep each separate.

BASIC BREADS/CEREALS UNITS

Any portion listed is a Unit. No other units are included (milk for your cereal or butter on your bread)

GIRLS: 6 Units a day, minimum   BOYS: 8 Units a day, minimum
Maximum calories: 360   Maximum calories: 480

A note of caution: There is no way you can ever be sure of the calories you're eating in any manufactured product (or in any food, since many variables influence the count). Manufacturers frequently change recipes and amounts of ingredients in standard items. In addition, there is enormous variation among brands of similar products.

Ounce for ounce, most commercial bakery breads are calorically similar. But a thinner slice or one with a lot of air holes will naturally have fewer calories. The same holds true for other types of breads, rolls, buns. So, once again, the stress is on variety. Don't get hipped on one thing.

The Breads/Cereals Units, like all Units except Milk, have been calculated to average out as long as you eat a variety of them. The idea is to maintain a weekly average of about sixty calories for each Breads/Cereals Unit. This gives you leeway in two directions. It doesn't give you *consistent* leeway to choose Units from the upper calorie range, however.

In general, Breads/Cereals means *all* cereals of any kind, all breads, crackers, whole grains, pastas, flours, and the listed vegetables.

You may use your discretion in making substitutions if you play detective with the calories. (No Cop-out substitutions, however!) If a package tells you one piece, or portion, has six calories, you can then use ten pieces as a substitute for some Breads/Cereals Units. Ten pieces will be calorically equal to sixty calories.

In lieu of knowledge gained from the label or from a convenient pocket-sized calorie counter, use the following as guidelines for food types in breads and cereals.

ABOUT THE BASIC DIET PLAN

	Average Calories		Average Calories
1 slice whole-wheat, rye, or enriched white bread	60	½ cup oysterettes (20)	60
½ English muffin	40	½ cup fresh lima beans (immature beans are very high in iron)	75
½ cup cooked cereal (corn meal mush, farina, grits, oats, oatmeal, cream of rice, rolled whole wheat, plain noodles)	70	½ cup sweet corn or 1 medium-sized ear of corn on the cob	85
⅓ cup cooked rice	60	½ cup parsnips	48
⅓ cup cooked spaghetti	56	1 small white potato, baked, with skin, or ½ cup mashed potato	70
¼ cup bran	47	1 small pancake	65
¾ cup ready-to-eat, unsweetened cereals (corn flakes, oat flakes, puffed rice, Wheaties, etc.)	60	½ small waffle	60
		1 bread stick	39
		⅛ cup bread crumbs	45
½ shredded-wheat biscuit	45	½ small biscuit	45
½ bun or roll for hot dog or hamburger	60	½ small breakfast muffin	60
2 graham crackers	55	1 slice Thomas' gluten bread	35
4 saltines	50	1 slice Thomas' protein bread	45

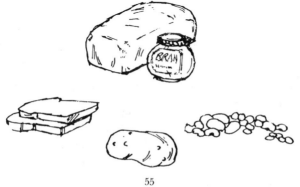

BASIC FRUITS UNITS

Any portion listed is a Unit. Canned juices must be unsweetened; canned fruits must be drained of syrup. Minimum daily allowance: 3 choices. One choice must come from the Vitamin C Group. Maximum calorie allowance: 175 (Unless you have extra calories to spare for the day).

The following are top-ranking Vitamin C fruits. Choose at least one every day:

	Average Calories		*Average Calories*
1 medium orange	70	½ cup orange juice (fresh, frozen, canned)	55
½ small grapefruit	70		
1 cup strawberries, fresh	54		
1½ oz. frozen strawberries	45	½ cup grapefruit juice (fresh, frozen, canned)	44
1 wedge honeydew melon (2" x 7")	49		
1 small guava, fresh (spectacular Vitamin C)	49	½ cantaloupe, about 5" in diameter. (Yellow-fleshed variety. Vitamin A winner, too!)	40
1 small mango (Vitamin A)	65		
2 medium lemons	40	½ small papaya (Vitamin A)	45
½ cup tangerine juice (fresh, frozen, canned)	45	1 large tangerine	45

Your other two choices may come from this list:

	Average Calories		*Average Calories*
1 small apple	70	½ cup fresh blackberries	40
½ cup apple juice (fresh, canned)	62	¼ cup canned blackberries	54
½ cup applesauce (unsweetened)	50	½ cup fresh blueberries	42
		3 oz. frozen blueberries (unsweetened)	52
2 medium apricots (fresh)	51	¼ cup canned blueberries	48
4 dried apricot halves	60	12 large cherries	60
3 medium apricot halves (canned)	75	½ cup canned cherries	61
		2 pitted dates	70
½ medium banana	60	2 small figs, fresh	60

	Average Calories		Average Calories
1 large fig, dried	55	½ cup pineapple juice	60
½ cup canned fruit cocktail	45	(fresh, frozen, canned)	
		2 medium plums,	50
½ cup (20) grapes	42	(fresh, canned, dried)	
¼ cup grape juice	56	2 large uncooked prunes	54
1½ large limes	52		
½ cup loganberries, fresh	45	¼ cup prune juice	42
2 medium nectarines	60	2 tablespoons raisins	54
1 medium peach, fresh	45	½ cup black raspberries, fresh	50
2 oz. frozen peaches	44		
2 canned peach halves	60	½ cup red raspberries, fresh	35
1 small pear, fresh	50	2 oz. red raspberries, frozen	52
2 canned pear halves	50	1 cup cubed watermelon	56
¾ cup pineapple, fresh	56	1 watermelon wedge,	55
1 slice canned pineapple	65	about ½" x 1" x 10"	

BASIC VEGETABLES UNITS

Any portion listed is a Unit. Vegetables may be fresh, frozen, canned, dried. Minimum daily allowance: 3 choices. No calorie restrictions on fresh vegetables. No other calorie restrictions, except as noted by the italics. Daily choice should include one iron-rich vegetable and at least one Vitamin C vegetable.

The following vegetables are top-quality sources of iron and frequently of Vitamin A as well. Starred items are also good sources of Vitamin C. All vegetables are cooked, unless otherwise noted.

	Average Calories	COMMENTS	Average Calories
* 1 cup beet greens	39	Excellent A, good C, and calcium	
* 1 cup broccoli	44	Unbeatable source of C, with good A, calcium, niacin	
* 1 cup chard	30	Unbelievable in A, good in C, calcium, and riboflavin. Top-rank winner in iron, too	
* ¾ cup collards	60	Another star with calcium, A, C, niacin, riboflavin	

57

	Average Calories	COMMENTS
* ½ cup dandelion greens	40	1 cup packs more than 5 times your Vitamin A needs for the day! Just the tops in iron
* 2 stalks fresh endive	25	A, C, calcium, and niacin
* 4 leaves escarole, fresh	20	A, C, calcium, and niacin
* ½ cup green peas	56	Great niacin, good C
* ½ cup garden cress	37	Top of the mark in iron
* 1 bunch watercress, fresh	20	A, C, calcium, and tops in iron
* 1 cup kale	44	Very high in A, good C, niacin, calcium, and protein
4 large mushrooms, fresh	16	Great niacin
1 cup canned mushrooms	30	
* 1 cup mustard greens	31	Excellent A, great C, good calcium
* 1 cup spinach	46	Excellent A and C
* ½ cup squash, winter	45	Very rich in Vitamin A, also
* 1 cup turnip greens	43	Smashing A, C, calcium, niacin

Other vegetables with high iron content are the dried beans and peas (which are treated as Protein Units) and fresh baby limas (a Breads/Cereals Unit). All of the foregoing list is notable for its Vitamin A content in addition to the iron. Other important Vitamin A vegetables (not necessarily as spectacular in iron) are:

	Average Calories
1 cup carrots, diced	44
2 medium-raw carrots	42
½ cup canned pumpkin	38
* 1 medium tomato, fresh	30
* 1 cup canned or fresh-cooked tomato	46
* 1 cup tomato juice	50

Some of the leafy vegetables on the list (chard, collards, kale, for instance) may be unfamiliar to you. Some are available fresh only in regions where they are popular. Ask the produce manager of the supermarket where your family usually shops when and if he ever stocks them. Often you can find them in the frozen foods section.

Dandelion greens should be picked when young, before they blossom.

ABOUT THE BASIC DIET PLAN

The vegetables on the following list, in addition to the starred ones listed on pages 57–58, are very high in Vitamin C.

	Average Calories	COMMENTS
1 cup cooked green beans	27	
½ cup cooked Brussels sprouts	30	Good iron, too
1 cup raw cabbage	24	Good calcium
1 cup cooked cabbage	40	
1 cup cooked Chinese cabbage	25	
1 cup raw cauliflower	25	More than a full day's C requirement
1 cup cooked cauliflower	30	
1 raw cucumber	25	
1 cup kohlrabi, fresh	40	A winner in Vitamin C
1 cup cooked kohlrabi	47	
8 pods okra	30	
1 medium onion	50	
1 medium green pepper, raw	16	Fabulous Vitamin C!
2 medium canned pimientos	20	Don't forget to include in your tossed salads.

Other vitamin- and mineral-rich vegetables:

Radishes, 1 medium	5	Dash of A, good C
½ cup rutabagas (yellow turnips), cooked	30	Good C
1 cup sauerkraut, canned	32	Calcium, C
1 cup turnips, cooked	42	Good C
½ cup beets, cooked	35	
1 cup summer squash	35	Good C
1 leaf lettuce	3	
1 large stalk celery	4	

White potatoes, a Breads/Cereals Unit, also have lots of C plus the B vitamins.

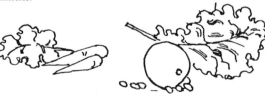

BASIC SOUP UNITS
Minimum weekly allowance: 5

All of the following are commercially prepared products. Home-made soups are usually a better nutritional choice, but you will have to figure approximate calories from ingredients in each individual recipe. Vegetable juices count as a Unit.

	Average Calories		*Average Calories*
1 cup of any bouillon: beef, chicken, vegetable	10	½ cup oyster, clam, fish chowder or stew prepared with water (if you prefer milk, use a portion of your Milk Unit rather than readjust calorie counts, or cut down the amount of soup or chowder)	70
1 cup of any broth : beef, chicken	25		
½ cup of any broth with rice or noodles	22		
½ cup bean soup	50		
½ cup any "cream of" soup prepared with water	40		
½ cup clear madrilène	20	½ cup tomato or vegetable	50
1 cup clear consommé	20	1 6-ounce glass of any canned tomato or vegetable juice	40
½ cup minestrone	50		
½ cup green pea soup, split pea	60		

13

THE BASIC DIET PLAN
IN ACTION

This is a general guide for daily food distribution. You may think up as many variations as you want, and you may need to adjust distribution to fit your schedule. Just stay within the Unit method and within your calorie allowance.

Daily Food Distribution

BREAKFAST
1 Fruits Unit
½ to 1 Protein Unit
1 Milk Unit
1 to 2 Breads/Cereals Units
1 Fats Unit

MID-MORNING SNACK
1 Milk Unit
1 Vegetables Unit
1 Breads/Cereals Unit

LUNCH
1 Protein Unit
1 to 2 Vegetables Units
2 Breads/Cereals Units
1 Fats Unit

MID-AFTERNOON SNACK
1 Fruits Unit
1 Milk Unit
1 Vegetables Unit, if
desired. (This is a good
place for boys to add
their extra protein and
Breads/Cereals Units)

DINNER
1 Protein Unit
2 to 3 Vegetables Units
1 to 2 Breads/Cereals
Units
(This depends upon
how many you have
already used during
the day)
1 Fats Unit
1 Milk Unit

EVENING SNACK
1 Breads/Cereals Unit or
alternate
1 Vegetables Unit
½ Milk Unit for boys
1 Fruits Unit

As you can see, there are many ways to distribute your food Units throughout the day. If you cannot manage a mid-morning snack, add part of the food to breakfast, part to lunch or either of the other two snacks. The distribution will depend on what you choose as your snack. For instance, you might want the Breads/Cereals Unit with breakfast and the Milk Unit with lunch.

If your dinner hour is customarily late, you may be better off having *two* snacks during the afternoon. Have a portion of your food at mid-afternoon and the usual evening snack food in late afternoon.

Boys should increase their Protein Units by an amount equal to three ounces of meat or poultry or four ounces of fish. Add Protein by (1) doubling either lunch or dinner portions, (2) splitting an extra Unit between morning and afternoon snacks, or (3) increasing both lunch and dinner portions somewhat.

Boys between thirteen and nineteen should increase their calcium intake by adding an extra half cup (minimum!) of skimmed milk each day to the basic allowance of one quart.

How to Design Your Own Menu

Get together with Mom on this one. You should be close collaborators on this part of the program.

Start by making a list for each day of the week from the Basic Units lists. Just write down a variety of foods you want to eat for the week—within financial reason, of course.

Follow the general diet plan for distributing your food over the day's time. The chart on pages 64–65 shows how a week's selection of food might be distributed.

After you've listed choices for the week in each food category, you may find some things that just don't go together. Trade them around. A Protein Unit you selected for Tuesday might go better with Friday's vegetable list. Or stick your Sherlock nose into a cookbook and see what you can concoct.

Keep menus simple at first. Fancy combinations come after you get the hang of things.

You can substitute canned or frozen vegetables and fruits for fresh ones. They are very similar nutritionally. Calorie counts are similar, too.

The Basic Units list of fruits shows you correct portions for canned fruits, drained of syrups. Few frozen fruits are obtainable without sugar, but when they are, you can make a one-to-one substitution.

Don't substitute canned or frozen vegetables in sauces or butter unless the label tells you the calorie content.

Note that the suggested food selections on the chart are for an 1,800-calorie plan. Boys add one Protein, one half Milk, and two more Breads/Cereals Units. Boys and girls both may have a maximum daily allowance of two teaspoons of sweets, such as honey, sugar, jams, syrups.

If one of your daily Protein Units is something other than beef, pork, or lamb, you may add one tablespoon of cottage cheese, pot cheese, or ricotta to your menu. Farmer's cheese, where available, is an excellent low-calorie, high-protein substitute for cottage cheese.

Use any of the above cheeses in a milk shake or as a butter replacement on a baked potato. Add chopped fresh chives or dill for a delicious change of pace.

	Proteins GIRLS (3) BOYS (4)	Breads / Cereals GIRLS (6) BOYS (8)	Fruits (3)
Monday	Eggs Chicken Meat Loaf	Toast Cereal Bread Breadstick	Canteloupe Apple Pear
Tuesday	Bacon Cottage cheese and eggsalad mix Swordfish	Waffle Graham crackers Saltines Corn-on-cob Oysterettes Bread	Mango Blackberries Plums
Wednesday	Egg Franks Veal	Toast Bun Rice Breadstick	Strawberries Banana Orange
Thursday	Cottage cheese Ham Sardines	Bread Saltines Cornbread Black-eyed peas	Canteloupe Apple Raisins
Friday	Sausage Roast beef Chicken	Cereal Toast Bread Graham crackers Saltines	Orange Peaches Pineapple
Saturday	Cheese Sole Steak	Cereal Toast Potato Oysterettes Bread	Blueberries Tangerine Prunes
Sunday	Cheese Pork chop Fish	Toast Noodles Lima beans Bread	Applesauce Strawberries Apricots

Milk GIRLS (4) BOYS (4½)	Vegetables (3)	Soups 5-A-WEEK	Fats (3)
4 cups	Asparagus Tomato juice Salad Squash Fresh vegetables Broccoli	Consommé	Butter* Mayonnaise Oil
4 cups	Vegetable juice Stewed tomatoes Salad Cauliflower Carrots Scallions	Vegetable soup Chowder	Butter* French dressing Butter*
4 cups	Cole slaw Kohlrabi Vegetable juice Salad	Soup	2 fats 1 nuts
4 cups	Salad Collards Green beans Radishes Carrots Assorted pickles	Broth	Mayonnaise Mayonnaise Butter*
4 cups	Salad Green peas Chard Sweet Potato Vegetable juice Salad	Soup	Butter* Mayonnaise Butter*
4 cups	Tomato juice Spinach Vegetable marinade Eggplant Carrots Tossed salad	Soup	Butter* Butter* Oil
4 cups	Turnips Sauerkraut Vegetable juice Salad Cauliflower Brussels Sprouts	Soup	Butter* Sour cream Butter*

* Margarine may be used
instead of butter

THE WEEK'S MENU

Here's how you might take your weekly list and turn it into a menu following the daily food distribution plan:

MONDAY

BREAKFAST

¼ cantaloupe   2 eggs, scrambled in Teflon pan
2 slices whole wheat toast, 1 teaspoon butter or margarine
1 glass of milk

SNACK

¼ cantaloupe   ¾ cup wheat flakes (1 teaspoon sugar)
1 glass of milk (part with the wheat flakes)

LUNCH

1 cup beef consommé
1 sliced chicken sandwich (3 oz. chicken, 2 slices enriched bread,
1 tsp. mayonnaise)
1 cup asparagus (Save the juice!)
½ cup tomato juice (canned)

SNACK

1 glass milk shake (with farmer's cheese. See recipe)
1 apple, small

DINNER

Dish of fresh vegetable appetizers: carrot sticks, celery,
cauliflower florets, pickles; cheese dip (see recipes)
Tossed salad: lettuce, spinach, tomato, green pepper slivers,
chopped onion, seasoning, oil/vinegar dressing
3 ounces meat loaf (see recipes)
½ cup acorn squash   1 bread stick   1 cup broccoli

SNACK

1 glass milk   2 canned pear halves, no syrup

TUESDAY

BREAKFAST

4 slices Canadian bacon   ½ cup blackberries with milk
(from allowance)
½ small waffle, 1 teaspoon butter,
1 teaspoon honey, jam, jelly, or syrup
1 glass milk

SNACK

1 small mango   2 graham crackers
1 cup asparagus juice

LUNCH

1 cup vegetable soup with 4 saltines
1 egg/cottage cheese salad (see recipe),
including lettuce, slices of tomato,
cucumbers, radishes, cress,
pickle
1 glass milk   1 slice whole-wheat bread

SNACK

large tossed salad: spinach, romaine, escarole,
½ small sliced onion,
seasoning, 1 tablespoon French dressing
1 glass milk

DINNER

1 cup New England style clam chowder
(made with skimmed milk)
½ cup oysterettes
4 ounces swordfish
corn on the cob
1 cup stewed tomatoes
1 teaspoon butter with lemon and seasoning for swordfish

SNACK

Carrot sticks, cauliflower florets, fresh scallions
1 glass milk   2 fresh plums

WEDNESDAY

BREAKFAST

¾ cup strawberries with 1 teaspoon sugar
2 slices French toast (1 egg, 2 slices enriched bread)
½ cup milk
1 teaspoon jam, jelly, syrup, or honey

SNACK

½ banana   ½ cup milk

LUNCH

½ cup black bean soup, ready-to-serve type (It's loaded with iron!)
2 frankfurters with mustard, relish, pickles
1 frankfurter roll   ½ cup cole slaw (see recipes)
1 glass milk

SNACK

1 small orange   1 glass vegetable juice (fresh/canned)
1 breadstick

DINNER

Tossed salad, mixed greens, lemon dressing
Veal stew (see recipe; allow 2 Fats Units)
⅓ cup cooked rice   1 cup kohlrabi   1 glass milk

SNACK

1 cup milk   6 small nuts

Note on Wednesday Lunch

If you're having cole slaw in a restaurant, you will use one Fats Unit for the mayonnaise in it.

Note on Thursday Dinner

This dinner was chosen to show you how typical regional food may be included in your diet, with only slight modification. A quick look at the Calorie Chart shows that black-eyed peas aren't as high in calories as other dried legumes. Here they are used with corn bread (the number of calories in one piece was calculated from the recipe) as two of the Breads/Cereals Units.

68

THURSDAY

BREAKFAST
1 glass vegetable juice
¼ cantaloupe with half of your cottage cheese Unit.
(Save other half to make your fresh vegetable dip.)
1 cup milk

SNACK
½ portion of apple/celery/raisin salad (see recipe)
on bed of lettuce (allow one Fats Unit for the mayonnaise)
1 glass milk

LUNCH
1 cup beef broth with 4 saltines
2 open-faced sardine sandwiches (2 slices enriched bread, 1
can of sardines, well-drained, 1 to 2 tablespoons
chopped onion, and 1 teaspoon mayonnaise)
Pickles (dill, cucumber, or sweet.
No need to limit quantity. All varieties are
low in calories.)
¼ cantaloupe

SNACK
½ portion of apple/celery/raisin salad, as above
1 glass milk

DINNER
(*See note on page 68*)
Tossed salad with lemon dressing
½ cup black-eyed peas (Southern style, see recipe)
3 ounces *lean* portion of ham   1 cup collards
1 cup green beans   1 piece corn bread 2″ x 2″ (see recipe)
1 teaspoon butter

SNACK
Fresh vegetables with cottage cheese dip
(carrot slivers, plum tomatoes, strips of green pepper)
1 glass milk

FRIDAY

BREAKFAST
1 glass vegetable juice (fresh) or 6-oz. can V-8
2 small pork sausage links, well-cooked and drained
½ cup oatmeal, 1 teaspoon sugar
1 slice toast, 1 teaspoon butter
1 glass milk

SNACK
1 small orange 1 glass milk 2 graham crackers

LUNCH
Roast beef sandwich (2 slices bread, 3 ounces lean
roast beef, mustard), pickles
Lettuce and tomato salad with 1 teaspoon mayonnaise
½ cup green peas
(add these, cold, to above salad if you pack a lunch to take
to school)
1 glass vegetable juice.

SNACK
1 glass milk with ½ cup fresh pineapple as milk shake (see
recipes)

DINNER
1 cup chicken noodle soup with 4 saltines
3 ounces baked chicken
Tossed salad with greens, cucumbers, onions, lemon dressing
1 cup chard
½ small sweet potato with 1 teaspoon butter

SNACK
1 glass milk
2 halves canned peaches, without juices

SATURDAY

BREAKFAST
2 slices whole-wheat toast
with 2 slices American cheese, sliced tomatoes
1 glass milk

SNACK
½ cup blueberries with 1 teaspoon sugar
¾ cup Wheaties   ½ cup milk

LUNCH
½ cup oyster stew
(frozen, prepared with water)
with ½ cup
oysterettes (20)
1 glass tomato juice
4 ounces baked sole with 2 butter Units, lemon
1 cup spinach   ½ cup carrots
1 small tangerine

SNACK
Vegetable marinade (see recipes)
1 slice gluten bread   ½ cup milk

DINNER
Tossed salad   3 ounces steak
1 small baked potato
with 1 tablespoon cottage cheese
Eggplant Creole
(see recipe section)
1 glass milk   2 medium prunes, fresh

SNACK
1 glass milk

SUNDAY

BREAKFAST

½ cup applesauce   2 ounces cheddar cheese
2 slices toast with 1 teaspoon butter, 2 teaspoons honey
1 cup milk

SNACK

¾ cup strawberries with 2 tablespoons sour cream

LUNCH

½ cup tomato soup with 1 slice rye bread with butter
1 lean pork chop with sauerkraut
1 cup turnips   ½ cup lima beans
1 cup milk

SNACK

4 halves dried apricots spread with
1 tablespoon ricotta cheese
1 cup milk

DINNER

1 glass vegetable juice
Tossed salad, 1 tablespoon lemon dressing
Tuna fish casserole (see recipes)
1 cup cauliflower with mushrooms/parsley sprinkled with
Parmesan cheese
½ cup Brussels sprouts

SNACK

1 cup milk   Fresh vegetables/cheese dip

Note on Snacks
Try any combination of the following for great snacking with the high-
protein cheese dip: radishes, carrots, small canned beets, tiny onions, pi-
miento strips, button mushrooms, cauliflower florets, green pepper sticks,
plum tomatoes, cold asparagus slices, cooked broccoli slices.

15

DIETING WITHOUT DILEMMA

There are dozens of favorite family dishes or meals that you can take part in with slight modifications and just a little attention to detail. If you follow the Basic Diet Plan and watch your portions and food distribution, you need not dismiss whole classes of foods from your regular diet.

Here are some suggestions for a few common dishes you can enjoy along with the rest of the family.

The New England Boiled Dinner

This traditional dinner need not be off limits. It's nutritious, mouth-watering, and needs very little variation to fit the system well. Here's what dieter and cook do:

THE HAM: Select for leanness ham that is fresh, cured, cooked, or canned. Trim all fat. You won't lose any flavor by removing it, contrary to what many people think. It's the meat that packs the flavor.

THE VEGETABLES: Add vegetables (except cabbage) to pot when meat is almost cooked. If it's a cooked ham to start with, put ham and vegetables in together at the start. Cook until carrots, potatoes, onions are almost done. Add cabbage wedges and continue cooking for another ten to fifteen minutes, or until cabbage is just soft and tender. Save the pot juices for soup.*

---

* If you use a teaspoon of caraway seeds and a generous pinch of tarragon, you will have a delicious, sweet juice (when chilled) for between-meal snacks.

Serve the dieter: 3 ounces lean ham (1 Protein Unit); 1 small potato (1 Breads/Cereals Unit); 1 small onion, 1 wedge (at least ¼) of cabbage, ½ cup carrots (3 Vegetables Units). Add to his menu a generous tossed salad, glass of vegetable juice, or glass of milk if milk is on the schedule. Dieter may use 1 Fats Unit for butter for cabbage and potato and 1 Fats Unit for salad dressing.

Approximate calories in the meal: 415 without the milk; 502 with it.

Or Would You Prefer Frankfurters and Beans?

Plan in much the same manner. But use both franks and beans as a Protein Unit. Divide the allotment: one frank plus a scant one half cup of beans gives you good protein and just clips the mark on calorie allowance: about 250. For the balance of your meal, add vegetables, other Units as you wish, according to your day's plan. There's no rule that says you *must* have two or three franks with a full plate of beans!

The whole trick to eating a balanced, calorie-controlled diet is to plan ahead, using the Unit system as a guideline to insure meeting nutritional needs. That's why a week's menu is really a necessity. If you *know* what you're going to eat, how much of it, then you also know how to plan for emergencies, how to swap, and how to save calories for special occasions.

The Seafood Dinner

It's a great dinner for important proteins and minerals. Just remember to turn down all fried seafoods (or the calorie counts will skyrocket!).

Plan ahead to save your Fats Units so you can have butter with that delicious baby lobster. You can also have a shrimp cocktail or clams on the half shell as a part of your Protein Unit with the lobster.

Or if you prefer baked fish, you might choose a clam broth for openers. If eating out, you'll order the baked potato (usually over-sized) and eat *half* of it unless you have saved two Breads/Cereals Units. Don't forget the tossed salad.

If it's a clambake, enjoy the clams, shrimp, and lobster,

but pass up the franks and sausage. One corn on the cob is allowed. You *did* plan for a Fats Unit of butter, didn't you? Enjoy as much of the broth as you want and as many vegetables.

A fruit for dessert (one Unit from your menu plan) is good for finishing touches.

Going Southern?

Yes, you can, and here's how.

Southern-fried chicken: One Unit as listed under Basic Protein Units. Rice is traditional, but remember that you eat one third cup, cooked, and you allow a Breads/Cereals Unit for it.

You've planned ahead, so you have a Fats Unit of butter or margarine for the rice. You'll pass up biscuit and corn bread, unless you are willing to trade the rice for them.

Turnip greens, green beans, tossed salad, fresh tomatoes —go ahead. (No vegetables cooked with salt pork or fatback, however!) No fried corn or fried okra. Save them for another time when you can fit in a fried food without tipping the calorie scales.

Here is a recipe for the classic Southern-fried chicken. You may use the same method for frogs' legs and pan fish.

SOUTHERN-FRIED CHICKEN

1 small, young chicken (called a "broiler" or "fryer," depending on the section of the country)
1 paper or plastic bag containing a cup or so of flour, seasoned well with salt and pepper (traditionalists prefer a paper bag)

The true Southern-fried chicken is the least expensive calorically. It isn't fried with bread crumbs, corn flakes, or batter, contrary to what many cookbooks may tell you. The secret to calorie-saving frying also lies in a very hot oil. It browns the food quickly before it can absorb too much grease.

Cut the chicken into small pieces. The Southern style of cutting up chicken gives an extra piece, called the "wishbone," but it isn't mandatory. Rinse chicken and let drain; don't wipe dry.

Heat a deep skillet of oil until piping hot. Oil should be

at least an inch deep; but preferably, if the skillet will hold it, the oil should be deep enough to cover the chicken.

Shake the chicken, a few pieces at a time, in the bag of seasoned flour until well-coated. Place chicken in the hot oil, using pincer tongs to avoid hot oil splashes. Brown lightly and quickly, on both sides, then turn down the heat somewhat. Don't put a cover on the pan, and take care not to turn the heat too low.

Fry until chicken is deep golden brown and crisp. Drain well and serve while hot.

Soul Food

Good nutrition and good eating. Here's how to translate a dinner menu to a dieter's delight, using the same approach as in the New England Boiled Dinner.

HAM AND BLACK-EYED PEAS

1 very lean piece of ham (1–2 pounds)	1 bay leaf, crushed
1 can of black-eyed peas, or 1 package frozen	1 stalk diced celery (optional)
1 small onion, chopped finely	1 clove minced garlic
1 small green pepper, chopped finely	1–3 pods crushed red pepper (depending upon how hot you want the dish)
½ cup beef broth	

Instead of the crushed pepper, you can use a dash of Tabasco sauce, to taste, just before cooking is completed.

Put ham in large dutch oven, and cover with water. Bring water to boil, simmer ham until tender. In a small skillet, bring the ½ cup beef broth to a brisk boil, lower heat, and simmer onion and pepper for five minutes.

Remove ham from dutch oven, pour off (but save!) liquid, leaving about 1 to 1½ cups for the peas. Add peas and other ingredients to the pot. Cook about ten minutes, uncovered, until peas (if frozen) are almost done; otherwise, until canned peas are hot. Taste, correct seasoning—this is when you add the Tabasco for spicy hot peas. Put ham back into pot with the peas and cover pot for a few minutes' more cooking.

Serve while hot. Dieter gets portions as shown on Thursday's menu.

The apple/celery/raisin salad is a traditional nibbler's dish. Here's how it's made:

APPLE/CELERY/RAISIN SALAD

1 small apple (1 Fruits Unit)	1 small stalk of celery
2 tablespoons raisins (1 Fruits Unit)	2 teaspoons mayonnaise (2 Fats Units)

Pare and dice apples in small pieces. Chop celery very finely. Toss ingredients together, mixing well. Add pinch of salt. Serve on bed of lettuce.

Like the Italian Style?

You will have to pass up most pasta dishes unless you count your portions carefully and allow Units correctly. Forget the breaded and fried dishes. The problem isn't calories as much as it is cutting the protein portion to save calories.

Ravioli and manicotti are both off limits for the time being. One piece may be anything from 80 to 170 calories! And you may not get enough protein to equal a minimum Unit before you've gotten too many calories.

Better forget the homemade lasagna. One small piece, about 4″ x 2″, packs in more than 700 calories! Even half a portion of this (and who can settle for that?) doesn't bring the calories down enough.

Approach spaghetti and meat balls with restraint. Spaghetti is the same as rice: one-third cup equals one Breads/Cereals Unit. Meat balls—you may have three ounces only. The sauce? One to one and a half Fats Units for the olive oil lurking therein.

Add to your meal two more vegetables (but not spinach or escarole fried in olive oil) and your Milk Unit, if scheduled. No garlic bread unless you've planned ahead for it in your Breads/Cereals and Fats allowances.

These are just a few examples to give you an idea of how you can adjust ordinary meals to fit your diet plan. You can enjoy hundreds of dishes as long as you use the Unit system for planning your menu.

Remember which food groups are low in calories and

high in good nutrition so you will be alert to sensible choices.

Frequently just knowing what's in a dish and having a fair idea of how it's prepared can help you. Veal Parmigiana, for example, begins with veal—a good calorie and protein buy. But when it's breaded, fried, and topped with another protein, cheese, plus a rich sauce—look out! That wonderfully nutritious slice of veal has turned into a wonderfully nutritious plate of excess calories.

The only way to have the best of both worlds is to cut your portions down to allow for the extra calories. But don't let the cutting down interfere with your Unit balancing for good nutrition.

What's for Lunch?

During the school year, lunches may present a harder problem than any other meal of the day. If you're close enough to go home, then have lunch at home when you first start your diet. You can fix either hot or cold lunches, and you won't be surrounded by nondieters.

If you must eat in the cafeteria, you probably have a good idea of the kinds of foods regularly served. Plan your menus to include these foods in correct Units. You may have a sandwich (choose from the list that follows) by allowing for two Breads/Cereals Units, one Fats Unit for the mayonnaise or butter, a glass of milk or vegetable juice, and a mixed salad. Some of your snack food may be added in at lunch if you don't have a mid-morning break.

You might get variety in lunches with salads (featuring the types of fillings that give you a Protein Unit) or cottage cheese, fresh fruits, and so on.

In many areas, school cafeteria dietitians understand the problems of dieters and offer special diet plates with total calories indicated. You'll have to learn to estimate foods Units because the breakdown won't have been made for you—just the number of calories.

What's for the Lunch Bag?

If you carry a lunch to school, standard items should be included in the lunch bag. These are the extra rations of fresh vegetables for munching and the high-protein vegetable dip, a thermos of milk, soup, broth, or vegetable juice (ideally, both milk and one other). The small cans of V-8 juice are good, nonbulky substitutes for a second thermos. You may also have a packet of mustard, catsup, or chili sauce. You may vary your food distribution slightly to accommodate your school schedule.

Since sandwiches, whether made at home or bought at the cafeteria, are the main lunch choices, here is a listing of "innards" you can plan for. Just remember that portions are to be measured accurately at home and should be honestly estimated at the lunch counter.

The Mixed Salads

Chicken salad ½ cup
* Deviled crab 4 tablespoons
Egg salad 4 tablespoons
* Lobster salad 4 tablespoons
Salmon salad ½ cup
Sardine salad 4 tablespoons
Shrimp salad ½ cup
Tuna fish salad ½ cup
Turkey salad ½ cup

* Seldom available at school cafeterias, but you may have your own leftovers from a feast at home.

Luncheon Meats

Bologna (4″ diameter) 2 medium thin slices
Liverwurst (3″ diameter) 6 very thin slices
Vienna sausage (canned) 8 sausages
Tongue 3 ounces (usually 2 medium-thin slices)
Ham, boiled 3 ounces
Roast beef 3 ounces
Fresh ham 3 ounces
Capicola 1½ ounces
Cervelat 2 ounces
Meat loaf 4 ounces
Minced ham 3½ ounces
Salami (cooked type) 2½ ounces

Sizes of luncheon meats vary so from one brand to another that you will just have to weigh slices until you learn about how much equals a portion.

Turkey rolls, pressed chicken, meats such as sliced roast beef and ham, and most smoked fish have about the same calories as similar protein meats of the fresh-cooked kind. You can have four ounces of the fish, three ounces of the meat and poultry.

Don't forget to allow a Fats Unit if you use mayonnaise or butter on your sandwich. You need not allow for it in the preceding mixed salads list since calories have been prefigured for you in the portions.

Add Extra Proteins

Add extra proteins to basic dishes whenever you can. Powdered skimmed milk, defatted wheat germ, cheese, and eggs are good protein sources and can be added to dozens of dishes. Wheat germ also gives you extra B vitamins, and it's rich in Vitamin E, now thought to be the "youth" vitamin. Lucky you, if it is, for you'll be getting plenty of it with the Basic Diet Plan.

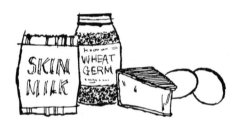

Here are a few ways of increasing protein in everyday dishes.

HIGH-PROTEIN MEAT LOAF
(protein, B vitamins, calcium)

1 lb. ground beef (have butcher cut out all fat before grinding)
¼ cup wheat germ
2 tablespoons skimmed milk powder
2 eggs
1 small chopped onion
½ medium green pepper, chopped
1 medium carrot, finely diced
1 small can chopped mushrooms with fluids (not butter-packed)
2 tablespoons chopped parsley
1 small can tomato sauce

Mix all ingredients except tomato sauce. Season to taste with: salt, pepper, thyme, garlic salt. If mixture seems too dry, add a tablespoon of water or vegetable stock. Shape into loaf and put into baking dish. Baste loaf with small can of tomato sauce; garnish with slices of onion. Bake in moderate oven (300–350 degrees) for about one hour, depending upon how thick the loaf is.

Calories: 222 per three-ounce portion.

HIGH-PROTEIN DIP/DRESSING
(protein, calcium)

Put one cup of skimmed-milk cottage cheese in the blender (215 calories, 44 grams of protein). Add two or three tablespoons of skimmed milk or evaporated skimmed milk for a smooth, creamy consistency. You will need a spatula to push the mix back down the sides, stopping the blender when necessary to break the air bubble.

Or use an electric beater or a hand-cranked egg beater; it will take a bit longer.

To make a sour-cream dip, add the juice of half a lemon.

Seasoning variation is endless. Try chives, dill, garlic salt, onion salt, celery seeds, poppy seeds, dried mustard, or seasoned salt—or anything you happen to be fond of. This dressing makes a great curried sauce with a dash of curry powder.

Farmer's cheese and skimmed-milk ricotta cheese are both good sources of extra, low-calorie protein and calcium. Try these cheeses on a serving of fruit or on a slice of toasted gluten bread.

HIGH-PROTEIN TOPPING
(protein, calcium)

2 tablespoons ricotta cheese (34 calories)   1 scant teaspoon honey (20 calories)

Mix together until creamy. Scandalously rich-tasting over berries, banana (half a small one is your Unit, remember?). Vary the flavor with a dash of nutmeg, cinnamon, or spice. If you've decided that one of your Fats Units for the day will be nuts, add six finely chopped almonds.

While we're on the subject of cheese, let's turn to a recipe for a milk shake. If it isn't quite sweet enough, add one teaspoon of sugar, jam, honey, or syrup (correctly measured, please!). This one is guaranteed to cure your mid-morning slump.

HIGH-PROTEIN MILK SHAKE
(protein, calcium, vitamins)

1 cup skimmed milk (1 Milk Unit) (87 calories)

1 Fruits Unit (apple, ½ banana, berries, pineapple—anything flavorful)

1 package of unflavored gelatin (30 calories)

2 tablespoons farmer's cheese, pot cheese, or ricotta (approximately 40 calories)

Put milk in blender. Turn to high, adding other ingredients slowly. Cut fruit in small pieces before you put it in so you won't jam the blender. To get a really thick, creamy shake, add a handful of cracked ice just before removing mix from blender. (Don't drop a whole cube in; you'll snap the blade off.)

Remember that you're adding the few calorie tidbits (the gelatin, cheese, etc.) on a day when you haven't chosen three meats as your Protein Units.

Cottage cheese and eggs seem to be meant for each other. Cottage cheese is really a dieter's dream—it's loaded with extra protein and calcium at little calorie expense. It can be combined with many foods for extra calcium and protein in dozens of different ways.

Try a breakfast combination with an egg. Scramble one egg in a Teflon pan. Just as the egg is done, quickly stir in two tablespoons of cottage cheese. Serve, sprinkled with fresh parsley or chives. Your calorie count? About 102, and you're getting full protein value. Cottage cheese has as much protein as the other egg from your daily Protein Unit. Meanwhile, you've saved 52 calories you can use for an extra piece of fruit.

HIGH-PROTEIN EGG SALAD
(protein, calcium, iron, Vitamin A)

Here's another way to combine cottage cheese and eggs for the lunch bag. Don't forget your thermos of vegetable juice and your slices of tomatoes and lettuce to go in the sandwich.

2 eggs, hard-boiled, chopped fine (154 calories; 1 Protein Unit)

1 tablespoon chopped green or red pepper (3 calories, Vitamin C and some A)

½ cup creamed cottage cheese (108 calories; ⅔ Protein Unit)

1 slice crisply fried, well-drained bacon, crumbled (50 calories; 1 Fats Unit)

1 tablespoon chopped onion (4 calories)

Salt and pepper to taste. Mix all ingredients well. Spread on sandwich bread. Enough for two healthy sandwiches: 158 calories each for the filling, 278 total with the bread. Boys may have two, the second being their extra Protein Unit. Girls, only one. Save the other for your kid sister (or your mother), who needs this great protein, too!

SHORT-CUT, HIGH-PROTEIN COLE SLAW
(protein, calcium, Vitamin C)
This is a quickie for the lunch bag or snack.

1 cup shredded cabbage (24 calories; 1 Vegetables Unit)
1 shredded carrot (21 calories; ½ Vegetables Unit)
⅓ to ½ cup high-protein vegetable dressing (75 calories, plus or minus ½ Protein Unit) Page 81.
1 tablespoon chopped onion (4 calories)

Toss cabbage, carrot, and onion together in large bowl with the vegetable dressing. If dressing isn't moist enough, add a teaspoon of ricotta or tablespoon of skimmed milk. Season with pepper.

Be a Calorie-Counting Sherlock

How ingenious can you get? Try your hand at cutting calories from ye olde traditionals! Sometimes simple substitutions can work wonders. Here's a case in point.

EGGPLANT CREOLE
Standard recipe: over 1,400 calories
New version: 304 calories

By substituting two slices of bacon for the usual ¼ pound of salt pork and 2 to 4 tablespoons of olive oil, the dish becomes much more sensible for the dieter.

1 medium eggplant (about 1½ pounds), pared and diced
2 slices bacon
1 medium onion, finely chopped
1 medium green pepper, finely chopped
2 cups canned tomatoes
1 small peeled garlic clove, whole (stick a wooden toothpick in it to rescue it later)
Dash cayenne pepper
⅛ teaspoon ginger
¼ teaspoon curry powder

Add salt to taste just before dish is ready to serve.

Fry the bacon crisply in a heavy Teflon skillet. Remove bacon and crumble; reserve. Pour fat out of skillet, but don't wipe the skillet. Sauté onions, peppers, with garlic clove and its identifying toothpick. When onions and peppers are just tender, add tomatoes, bacon, seasoning, and simmer for about half an hour, uncovered. Remove garlic clove after fifteen minutes unless you enjoy the gusto; if so, leave it in the full time.

Add pared, diced eggplant, and mix the whole batch well. Cook, uncovered, another half hour or until eggplant is tender. Makes about four servings. (If mixture should evaporate too quickly during last half hour, cover the pan awhile.)

WEDNESDAY NIGHT'S QUICK VEAL STEW

Note that the stew meat, onions, and peppers are not sautéed in 4 to 6 tablespoons of oil. Nor is the meat first rolled in flour; nor is any bacon fat added. Yet it's still a savory, hearty dish. And it's easy enough for you to whip up in no time.

1 to 1½ lbs. veal cubes (about 1"), very lean (785 calories)

1 can Franco-American mushroom gravy (150 calories)

1 medium onion, cut in half slices (50 calories)

½ medium pepper, chopped, not too finely (16 calories)

1 tablespoon parsley

½ cup broth or bouillon

1 small bay leaf

1 cup carrots, sliced (use frozen, if it's easier. Let them thaw in the lower part of refrigerator while you're off at school or work) (40 calories)

1 4- or 6-ounce can button mushrooms with juice (30 calories)

If you like a more highly seasoned gravy, try your hand at jazzing it up with 1 to 2 pinches of oregano, two pinches of ginger, a light sprinkling of dried orange peel, ½ tablespoon (or more if you like it) of curry powder. If you use the curry powder, add two tablespoons of white vermouth.

Use a heavy Teflon skillet with a lid that fits tightly. Bring broth to a full, rolling boil, add onions and pepper, and cook over reduced heat until tender. Add the veal chunks and cook just long enough to brown lightly. Add other ingredients. Cook for twenty to thirty minutes, depending on how much you've made, with cover on. Remove cover for final ten minutes of cooking to let some of the moisture evaporate. (If you add the suggested seasonings, do so when you put the gravy and other ingredients in.) The vermouth, incidentally, will evaporate, leaving only a subtle flavor blend with the curry.

Serve with cooked rice or noodles.

The dieter gets ⅓ cup of rice or ½ cup of plain noodles together with 2 tablespoons of gravy, three ounces of meat. Total calories in the veal stew: 1,071. Dieter's share: approx. 250.

Those Divine Concoctions

Be wary of that product of cooking genius, the casserole. Your best bet is one-half cup unless you know what's in the dish and can figure the calories.

The main idea behind a casserole is to stretch the food rations and food money. In devising ways to save while pleasing the palate, cooks have relied heavily on high-carbohydrate fillers, such as rice and noodles. With a fine sauce, these casseroles are a gourmet's dream but very caloric.

Even the nutritious, protein-rich bean casseroles are loaded with calories. Treat them as a Protein Unit: you may have three quarters of a cup, no more. The same quantity is usually safe for the meat types.

The following recipe is for a traditional tuna casserole; but as originally devised, it is inadequate in protein. One serving within your calorie allowance wouldn't give you enough protein. The only answer is to add more so that the net result is more protein for every calorie.

TUNA CASSEROLE
(protein, iron, calcium, spectacular niacin)

2 cups cooked noodles (replacing traditional 3 to 4) (214 calories)

½ cup canned green peas, drained (save the juice) (72 calories)

2 cans (7-oz. size) tuna, well-drained (double the usual 1 can) (784 calories)

1½ ounces cheddar cheese (many recipes don't call for the cheese) (160 calories)

1 can condensed mushroom soup (10½-oz. size) (80 calories)

1 tablespoon butter (100 calories)

½ cup mushrooms, stems and pieces (save the juice) (14 calories)

Optional seasoning: Worcestershire sauce, teaspoon sherry, dash of curry.

Drain noodles well. (Don't rinse, or you'll wash away the nutrients.) Toss with the butter to get them well-coated. Break up the tuna into chunks—don't shred. Toss all ingredients together, except the cheese.

Grate half the cheddar into the ingredients and mix well. Salt and pepper to taste. Oil a baking dish very lightly. Spoon in the mixture. Grate balance of cheddar over the top. Bake in hot oven (450 degrees) until top is brown and crispy. Serves five. Approximately 285 calories per serving.

LUSCIOUS LIVER

Lightly grease a Teflon pan—just enough to make it shiny. Put it on over high heat. When pan is hot, place two thin slices (about one-fourth inch thick) of liver, six inches by three inches, in the pan and sauté them quickly for three minutes, no more, on each side. Liver should be pink inside as is a good piece of rare roast beef. Serve immediately.

Rules of the Road

Plan ahead. Good planning is more than organization. It's always looking ahead and keeping the long-range goal in mind.

Make *every* calorie do its nutritional work. Think of the Cop-out Calories as deadbeats that don't pull their load.

Get in the tossed-salad habit. Mix different types of greens together. Experiment all you want. Make it a rule to eat at least one large tossed salad every day.

Look over the Vegetables Units and see the tremendous number of vitamins and minerals you get from those salad leaves. Add cucumbers, plum tomatoes, capers, seasonings. Use simple, noncaloric salad dressings, such as lemon juice mixed with a little water and loaded with herbs and spices. You get a Vitamin C booster in the lemon juice, too!

Soups are important, and the Units list shows you which of the canned ones and what quantities are on your diet. Homemade soups, meat and poultry broths and consommés, are naturals for extra vitamins and minerals. Add wheat germ to the pot for the extra B vitamins, protein.

Do as the professional runners do—rely on a cup of soup or broth as a quick energy pickup.

Remember that variety is always your keynote, for both calories and nutrients.

ACTION!

Now you know how tailoring menus to your needs makes pounds and inches disappear, but do you know exercise works a potent *mental magic* to make a new you?

The experts have come out with some startling findings. A good, well-rounded exercise program causes exciting changes in your personality and in your *academic performance.*

The New You

What are the personality changes? The biggest one is an improved self-image. Your whole attitude toward yourself changes. You feel and think differently. You become less depressed, less wrapped up in your own problems. Minor problems begin to melt away, and major ones start to look as if they can be solved.

Exercise gives you new zest for living—you look and feel better, and *you know it! Knowing* it is the key point. It makes for a happier you on the inside and a more radiant, cheerful, outgoing you on the outside.

And exercise pays dividends in the intellect department. It doesn't increase your intelligence, but it does *improve your mental performance.* Because exercise makes you more alert and more receptive, you use your mental equipment more efficiently. This means that better physical fitness can raise your grade averages and help stimulate your interest in subjects you thought you couldn't understand.

Aerobics, or Give Us Air!

A good exercise program begins within. It builds the all-important oxygen delivery system: a good heart, good lungs, and good blood vessels. It gets deep down to the powerful inner muscles and steps up the flow of rich, oxygen-laden blood.

Body cells need oxygen to burn food for energy and to build, repair, and maintain body tissues. A strong, efficient delivery system takes oxygen to where the action is and carries off combustion waste. It's your best health insurance for life.

The only exercises that can *consistently develop the oxygen delivery system are the aerobic exercises. (Aero* means air.) In short, they build a strong pump (heart), an efficient filter (lungs), and a good, clean pipe system (arteries and veins).

The top aerobic exercises for individuals are jogging, swimming, biking.

Good team or partner aerobics: squash, handball, basketball. Intense sports such as tennis, football, baseball, are great sports but don't qualify as true aerobics. They are "spurt" sports with much idle time between spurts. The object of aerobics is to get the *whole body moving and keep it moving.*

For most, jogging should be the basic choice. It requires no money or equipment and can be done anywhere and in any weather since you can do it at home. Indoors or out, you get the same benefits.

What's the Payoff?

You already know the most important one—the NEW you. Let's look at the others:

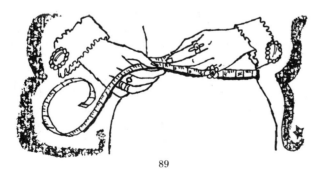

THE INCHES: Usually fewer inches are the first results to show up. The reason is simple. Exercise tones and tightens flabby muscles, and a slimmer you is reflected quickly in waistline, hips, and thighs. For the *underactive* teen-ager, results can be startling and dramatic in just a few weeks' time.

THE POUNDS: The object is to shave the *fat* pounds gradually, not the growing pounds. Your pound loss will depend upon the amount of food you eat, the amount of vigorous exercise you get, and your growth rate. Time is your best friend and most valuable ally. There are solid reasons why:

> —a weight loss program is a new way of life;
> —the Siamese triplets (remember them back on page 7?) need a chance to readjust to the new way;
> —a regular program of exercise steps up your metabolism and helps stabilize your weight at a *lower level.*

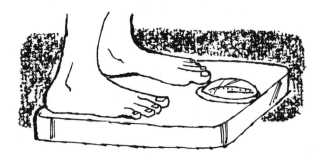

Once you stabilize at a lower level (and continue the exercise habit), even an increase in calories won't put the weight on as it did when you were inactive.

Where's the Fat?

Most is just under the skin (subcutaneous). The drawings on page 91 show you where the fat is in male and female. Because they're so visible, these are the areas where your major problems lie.

Normally, fat cells are small and oval-shaped. When you gain extra weight, the body stores excess fat, and the cells swell up like little balloons. Scientists have found that the more often you lose and regain weight, the more efficient the fat cells become. This is one reason why people regain weight faster as they get older. In effect, the fat cells are well-rehearsed in the up-and-down cycle.

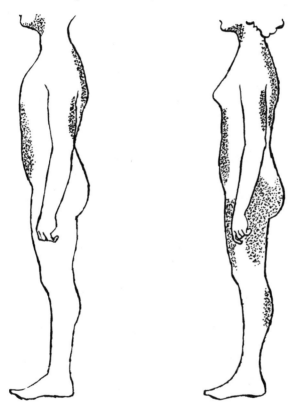

Spot Reducing

There's no such thing. Nothing can take the fat off in one spot only. When you lose weight, all fat cells discharge a minute amount at the same time all over the body. As you continue losing, the cells continue discharging fat until there is no more in storage. (The exact opposite occurs when you gain weight.)

So-called "spot reducing" is an illusion, at best. What actually happens is that exercise tightens and tones flabby muscles (*if* they're flabby—if not, it has no effect * except to keep muscles taut and healthy). The less flabby the muscle, the smaller and tighter it becomes, resulting in loss of inches but not loss of fat.

Part of the spot reducing illusion is due to the fact that we have more fat cells at certain spots than at others. Naturally, the proportionate decrease would *seem* bigger in the areas where fat cells are more numerous.

Happily, there's nothing wrong with reducing the inches as long as you know what you're losing. Pages 111–115 show you exercises for tightening muscles at specific trouble points.

* There are muscle-building exercises that increase both muscle mass and inches, but they aren't called "reducing" exercises.

17

TIPS FOR WINNING THE GAME

Keeping Your Records

Keep a daily diary of everything you eat and how much of it. Look up calorie counts and jot them down as soon after eating as possible, before you forget. Many overweights conveniently "forget" foods eaten after dinner, for instance. Since they never show up in the diary, the dieter can't understand why he isn't losing weight properly.

List *everything* you eat and drink at any time of day or night. If anything has calories, it counts.

Keep a daily activity record of your exercise. By comparing the two records, you can always figure out where your trouble is when your program isn't working. You always know when to cut back calories, or to add them, and when to increase energy output.

Special Instructions for Those Who Are Twenty or More Pounds Overweight

Before you begin a weight loss program, take a week's survey of both food intake and energy output. The Personal Survey Chart shows you how.

Your actual caloric intake may not be above normal range. In that case, your program should stress activity more than diet. Just double check your diet to be sure it's nutritionally balanced. Use the Basic Diet Plan as your guide.

Take your Personal Survey Chart with you when you go for your doctor's okay. He can advise you on adjusting your program to fit your special needs.

PERSONAL SURVEY FOOD CHART

Amount of food eaten	number of calories	Time of Day
total for day:		

PERSONAL SURVEY CHART: *PART ONE*

Instructions: Copy the chart into your diary, allowing a page for each day of the week.

List everything you eat and drink (except water). Enter the amount of food eaten in the left-hand column. In the center column, enter the number of calories, and in the right-hand column, the time of day. Add up total calories for each day, then the total for the week. Divide by seven to get your average daily caloric intake.

Look the chart over carefully. Are you "bunching" your calorie intake at certain hours? Do certain foods keep reappearing every day or several times a day? What kinds of foods are supplying the major portion of your calories?

How does your calorie intake compare to the recommended daily average from the Height/Weight Chart on pages 12–13?

If you're getting excess calories, you have trimming to do. You're probably eating a high proportion of fats and carbohydrates. Check the Basic Diet Plan and readjust your food balance.

If your average caloric intake is normal or lower and you're not losing weight, your energy level is much too low. Go to the second half of the chart to find the trouble.

PERSONAL SURVEY ENERGY CHART

Time of Day From: To:	Very Light	Moderate	Vigorous
Total			

a. m. / *p. m.*

PERSONAL SURVEY CHART: *PART TWO*

Instructions: Copy the chart into your diary, allowing one page for each day of the week.

Any energy output level depends upon how vigorously you do something. The three groupings are based on an assumed "normal pace." But there's a limit to energy increase. You can't parlay a sock-knitting session into a vigorous activity unless you knit a sock while climbing a mountain.

Check off your activity and record the amount of time spent at it in the appropriate column. Total the columns at the end of the day to see your typical daily pattern. After seven days, add ONLY the totals of the Vigorous Energy Levels. Divide by seven. The result is your average daily output.

Three hours of VEL means you're doing great! Your overweight problem probably stems from overeating or overemphasizing the wrong kinds of foods.

Less than a three-hour daily average indicates a probable underactive level. Just *how* underactive will vary, but if you score less than two hours daily, you need to change your schedule drastically. Get on the ball!

Give yourself credit for time spent at outdoor chores such as mowing the lawn. Walking behind a mower, particularly pushing it vigorously, is an energy output that counts. Rate most outdoor chores under "moderate" unless you really zing into them with vigor.

Energy Level Activities

Group One: Very Light Energy Level Activities:

Dressing or undressing

Driving a car

Many household tasks: dusting, sweeping, light cleaning, ironing

Sewing, knitting

Playing the piano, or almost any other musical instrument

Sitting, eating, studying, sleeping, resting, standing around

Strolling

Typing, writing

Group Two: Moderate Energy Level Activities:
    Walking at moderate speed (3 m.p.h.)
    Golf
    Ping-pong
    Moderate biking, lazy swimming
    Dancing (unless it's vigorous; you must be the judge)

Group Three: Vigorous Energy Level Activities:
    Swimming
    Running
    Jogging
    Very brisk walking
    Tennis (singles or mixed doubles in a foursome with good players)
    Most aerobic sports such as handball, squash
    Sawing, chopping wood

(If you do something that isn't on the lists, try to compare it in energy expenditure to something similar on the list so you can rate it properly.)

Part Two of the Personal Survey Chart will show clearly if you're spending the biggest part of your day in low-level activities.

Your usual day should break down into about eight hours of sleep, five to thirteen hours of light activity (including mealtimes, studying, school), and three hours of vigorous activities. Include gym classes if they're active.

Compare energy level outputs with calorie intakes. Both should give you a good idea of where to put your emphasis.

Cut Out the Cop-outs

Go over your list of foods eaten for the week and circle all the Cop-out Calorie Foods (these are listed in the Habit Profile questions). How many extra calories do the Cop-outs account for?

Every circle on the chart means a chance to trade a Cop-out for a food on your Diet Plan list.

Emergency Supplies

Always keep a supply of food on hand for beating the whammies.

In the refrigerator you should have fresh or canned fruits, ready to eat; plenty of raw vegetables, washed and ready to eat; a jar of vegetable juices; small cans of V-8 juice; thin slices of meats and cheese for high-protein nibbles.

In the cupboard you should have canned vegetables, canned fish, fruits, pickles, fruit juices, mushrooms—anything on your diet list. But keep in mind your portions.

Most vegetables, fresh, frozen, or canned, are unlimited as to portions permitted, and they are great appetite quenchers.

Take time to prepare foods beforehand for snacking. It's much easier to resist temptation when snacks are ready for eating. Otherwise, you're too tempted to grab a handful of Cop-out Calories.

SLIMMING DOWN

How did you rate your activity level on the Habit Profile Sheet? What did it actually turn out to be on the Personal Survey Chart? Was there a big discrepancy, or were you close?

If you're *honestly* in the normally active group, your first move is to correct diet patterns and food choices. Chances are, you can shave the extra pounds by cutting the Cop-out Calories and stepping up your daily activity.

The energy output spread between the inactive overweight and the active normal-weight can be enormous. The inactive teen-age boy, for instance, may be using only 2,500 calories a day while his counterpart may be burning up the turf frequently at 5,000–6,000! The same relationship exists for girls, usually at a lower level.

Your Basic Exercise Units

The exercise plan is similar to the Diet Plan. You build on a basic unit. Exercise units can be increased in two ways: by extending the time and by increasing the intensity of your activity.

Your exercise goal has two parts: the first is to increase gradually your physical fitness to peak level. The second is to meet your weekly minimum energy expenditure levels on a *regular schedule.*

Minimum Levels

Bear in mind that the exercise programs are MINIMUM LEVEL programs. They do not include any other activities in which you are (or should be!) involved. A teen-ager will have at least three hours of high-level activity a day, including gym class, *if* his or her program is active. Unfortunately, some teen-agers who don't take part in team or competitive sports aren't engaged in programs that are active enough.

As you get into your program and begin to shape up, look around for every opportunity to get more exercise. Talk to your gym teacher, and see if you can use the gym facilities during slack hours. Get some of your friends involved in your jogging, biking, or swimming activities.

There are thousands of jogging clubs throughout the country. Find out if there's one you can join in your community—or organize your own as lots of overweight teen-agers have done.

Competition is not the object of the exercise plan. You're not trying to outstrip or "beat" someone else or set a record. Build your program gradually to get yourself in shape. As you become better physically fit, you will automatically increase your output and fall into a rhythmic pattern uniquely your own.

Don't overstrain out-of-condition muscles. You won't get results any faster, just sore muscles.

If you can easily meet the beginning minimum weekly goals, move to the next level. (For instance, if thirty minutes is a snap, move to forty-five, and so on.) As soon as your level becomes comfortable, increase your time again. You will be a real winner if you can comfortably fit in a minimum of two hours of aerobic exercises every day!

You may choose from three basic aerobic exercises, or you may use any combination. Jogging was chosen for the module because it's free to everyone at any time. You may want to substitute swimming or cycling instead, if you have a pool or bike available to you. The important thing with all three is doing them on a regular schedule.

None of the aerobics will build bulging muscles. Instead, they slim and firm legs, trim ankles and waistline, help reduce hips and flatten tummies. They strengthen the powerful long, lean muscles in the legs and torso to give you the slim look.

Jogging and swimming, particularly, will redistribute

body fat so that you may actually drop down to a smaller size even before you have any significant weight loss!

In addition to the great slim look, you get to the immensely important oxygen delivery system—where real physical fitness begins!

Jogging

It isn't running. And it isn't walking. It's a slow, regular trot, somewhere between a fast walk and a run.

For instance, you can *walk* a mile in about fifteen minutes, so that kind of pace wouldn't be a jog. If you covered a mile in less than seven minutes, you would be *running*. You might say that a slow, beginner's jog would take twelve minutes for one mile. By the time you reach comfortable peak condition, you should be able to do thirty minutes of steady jogging at seven to eight minutes per mile without taking a break.

Thirty minutes is your MINIMUM BEGINNING basic aerobic module every day. If you're out of condition and can't do the entire half hour at one time, break it into segments until you get yourself in shape. Try two 15-minute, three 10-minute, or six 5-minute spans throughout the day.

This schedule will give you three and a half hours of aerobic exercises a week in the beginning. It moves into a minimum maintenance level of seven hours a week (and *that's* minimum for any teen-ager!).* All other exercises are add-on's for bigger payoffs sooner, or they're boosters you do each day.

If you drop out of your program for a while because of illness or some other problem, don't start in again at the old level. Reduce your minimum time, or break it up into segments throughout the day until you're back in shape.

Jogging Technique

(Use the same principles for swimming or cycling.)

If you've been underactive, start slowly without overtaxing yourself. Build up gradually to a peak performance level.

---

* You should be getting *at least* another daily hour of vigorous exercise (work or play), preferably a total of three hours daily for top performance.

Begin with a few minutes of slow, easy jogging. Then walk for a few minutes. Jog again. Alternate back and forth between jogging and walking in about equal segments.

If you're gulping air after the first half minute or so, your pace is too fast. Ease off and find your natural body rhythms. Never strain. You're building *endurance,* not speed.

Always take a few minutes of warm-up exercises before jogging. They make it much easier.

Those who are really out of condition and must break up the half hour into segments may prefer to do their shaping up indoors for the first month. The standing run pace is given along with jogging paces below.

Don't let bad weather interrupt your program—do it indoors! And *every single day,* after the first week. Remember that even five minutes six times a day equals a daily output of thirty minutes.

An Experiment to Charge the Inner Man

Your first warm-up experiment on page 21 was to help you begin developing your sense of self-awareness, and it emphasized your eating awareness. This second experiment will help to reinforce your new self-image and get you used to the idea of being really active and with it.

EXPERIMENT No. 2

MINIMUM TIME: three minutes
BEST TIME TO PRACTICE: just before you drift off to sleep or immediately after you awaken in the morning.

Picture yourself in your mind's eye as active, lively, and burning up lots of energy. Paint a complete mental image of yourself jogging, swimming, or cycling. Imagine what you're wearing and where you're exercising.

Develop the whole scene as clearly as if you were watching a movie. Try to capture the *inner feeling* of the activity, just as *if you were actually doing it.* Feel the powerful reaction of the deep inner muscles as they respond to the surge of fresh oxygen; feel the tingle of circulation awakening the muscles to the glow of action.

Mentally rehearse the picture while you capture the inner feeling.

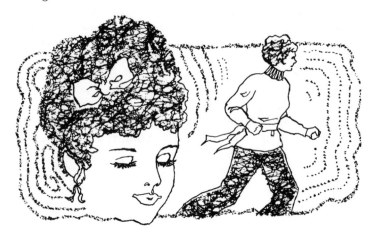

After you practice this experiment a few times, you'll do it easily and be amazed at the response you'll get from the inner man!

Gauging Your Physical Fitness

Aerobics should be fun and a challenge to you. There are no specific requirements such as 220 yards in X number of seconds. Your only basic module is time.

Allow your own natural rhythms to set the correct pace. As you become more physically fit, you will get so much fun from your energizing exercises that you will automatically *want* to increase your output.

If you try to "speed it up" beyond your level of the moment, you will tire and drop back to a lower level until you're ready to move up.

Within three weeks from the start of your program, you should begin to see definite changes—in the way you feel, in your weight, and in your size.

For the Technical-Minded

For those who feel they need guidelines, here are the general pacing ranges behind the three aerobics:

JOGGING: beginning pace, about twelve to thirteen minutes for a mile. Gradually moves upward over a period of six weeks to two months to about seven to eight minutes to the mile. (To determine a mile, pace it off. Your stride is about three feet, and 440 strides equal one fourth mile. So four laps of 440 strides become a mile.)

STANDING RUN: begins at eighty to ninety steps per minute. Increases to any comfortable, nontiring pace for thirty minutes minimum.

BIKING: begins at rate of five minutes for one mile; gradually works upward to minimum of two and one half minutes for one mile. Ideal is a steady but fairly vigorous pace for thirty minutes minimum without stops.

SWIMMING: begins with twenty-five-yard overhand crawl in eight minutes; works up to four minutes minimum. Continue workout for thirty minutes.

Add-On Exercises

These include warm-up exercises plus exercises for flexibility and shaping up. Do the add-on's every other day, gradually increasing to daily workouts.

Select a minimum of three warm-ups, two flexibility, and two figure-shapers. You can add to your basic module by increasing the number of times for each exercise or by increasing the number of exercises.

Gradually add in other daily activities to get yourself up to a minimum level of two hours a day.

How the Boosters Work

The object is to s-t-r-e-t-c-h your creative imagination and challenge your ingenuity. Boosters should be *your own ideas.* They can be as crazy or as silly as you want to make them.

Boosters are for the Mental Man—they put him to work reinforcing your goals and keeping you alert to your body movements. They increase self-awareness and help you to realize how and when you're being underactive.

Boosters are any exercises you can think up for use during the day to remind you of your new way of life. They keep mind and body in constant, close touch so that each reinforces the other.

Here are examples that other teen-agers have used. But the whole idea is for you to think up your own. Grab every opportunity, even if only for a few moments, to throw in a booster.

—Do deep knee bends while waiting for the elevator or when riding the elevator alone—one knee bend for each floor.

—Jog any time, anywhere, when you find yourself just standing around. Or jog-run from one place to the other instead of walking, say, from the bedroom to the living room.

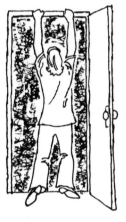

—Climb stairs instead of using the elevator.

—Don't catch the bus on the corner. Catch it at a stop a block or two farther along the route, and increase the distance you walk each day.

—Whenever you pass through a door frame, stretch up, in a long and lazy manner, grab the overhead lintel, and hang passively for a few moments.

Now—how many dozens of little ways can YOU think of to increase your energy output and remind yourself of what you're up to? Put your imagination to work, and see what you can come up with on your own. Your MINIMUM number of boosters is six a day—NOT six times, but six different TYPES.

Great Thought for the Day

An extra hour or two of activity per day will cause a spontaneous leveling off in your food intake. It sometimes causes an actual decrease! And it usually takes less than three weeks for you to see a difference.

So it's one more thing to look forward to in your new way of life.

19

THE ADD-ON EXERCISES

The times given are minimum. To get your full fifteen minutes of add-ons, either increase the number of times you do an exercise or use more exercises.

The Warm-ups

You may recognize a few of these. Some are old standbys, easily remembered, which have proved effective.

TOE TOUCHER

(You get flexibility with this one.) Stand erect, feet slightly apart, hands straight up overhead, overlapping. Now bend down and swing hands toward outside of right foot. Re-

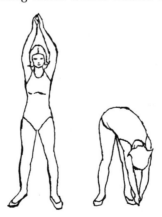

turn to erect position and repeat, bending to left foot. Four count: bend, up, bend, up. Boys: ten times; girls: six or more.

THE SWIMMER

Great for battery charging, loosening the shoulders. Stand with feet slightly apart. Bend forward at waist and do a swim-. mer's overhand crawl. Boys: one minute; girls: work up to one minute.

CHICKEN WINGS

Stand straight, elbows bent, hands loosely in front. Now rotate shoulder blades, pulling them forward, then circling back until shoulder-blade wings touch. You'll have to move those elbows and arms in a grinding motion. One minute in one direction, then rotate one minute in opposite direction.

HEAD SWIVEL

Stand straight, feet slightly apart. Drop chin into chest, then roll head around in large circle. Four times in one direc-

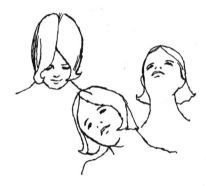

tion; four in the other. Keep body relaxed, feel gentle pull of neck muscles as head rolls.

SIGNALS

Stand erect, feet well apart. Raise arms shoulder high, out straight on each side like airplane wings. Swing forward in large circles ten times. Reverse, ten times.

Flexibility Exercises

These are the benders, stretchers, and twisters, but all are good for tightening muscles while getting you supple.

DANGLER

Spread feet about two feet apart. Hands straight up overhead. Now bend over, keeping knees straight, and let hands, arms, and torso hang limply. Bounce gently five times.

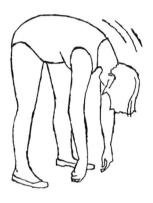

BENDER

Stand erect, with feet about a foot or so apart, hands at sides. Bend toward left side, sliding left hand down side of leg as far as possible. Raise right arm slowly and loop overhead,

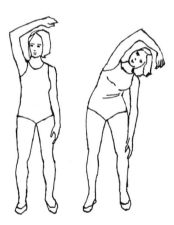

hand pointing limply down to left. Return to upright position and repeat in opposite direction. Do this five times each way.

TWISTER

This one's great for trimming your waist, too. Stand erect, feet slightly apart. Raise arms out to side, with wrists limp. Rotate torso from waist letting arms fling themselves in direction of rotation. Keep hips facing forward. Alternate direction of swing, but keep it loose and gentle. This one's deceptive, so don't get too vigorous.

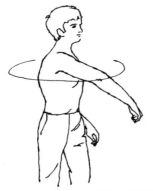

LONG MUSCLE STRETCHER

Sit on floor, legs as wide apart as comfortable in V. Keep knees straight. Bring hands together in front and slide them forward slowly along floor, letting torso bend forward to follow. Bounce gently. Return to sitting position. Place hands on top of thighs; slide them forward down top of legs, bending torso to follow. Return to sitting position, and repeat first

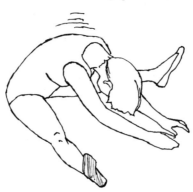

figure. Alternate back and forth, five times for each figure. Pause a moment between each figure.

BACK BENDER

Lie prone on your stomach, hands stretched out flat on the floor above your head. Put head back while pushing shoulders up. Bring feet back as if to touch head, knees bending. Gently does it; you grow into this one. Five times, NO MORE, at the start.

Trimming Your Sails

All these exercises give you a number of pluses but are particularly effective for building muscles and trimming inches in trouble spots.

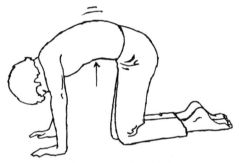

BACK AND STOMACH

Down on all fours. Let head hang down loose. Tighten stomach and backside muscles, making back arch like that of a cat; hold for five counts, but TIGHT. Relax. Now, do the opposite: thrust shoulders and head back, stomach downward

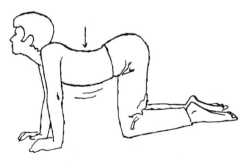

like that of a swayback horse; hold for five counts, TIGHT. Once a day is all.

FOR THE BACK

Stand beside a chair, one hand touching for balance. Swing outer leg backward, upward, with toe pointing outward like a dancer while body bends forward to "give" with the movement. Boys: ten times each leg; girls: seven times each leg. (In addition to back benefits, this one's good for fat bottoms and outer thighs.)

BACK, BUTTOCKS, WAIST, THIGHS

Before you get up from all fours, try this one. Raise right leg and extend it out to right as far as possible, point toe. Then swing back to the left as far as possible. Repeat with the left leg. You can watch the action if you want to. Five times per leg. Boys can start with eight.

WAIST, SHOULDERS, NECK

Don't get up; flop over on your back, arms stretched out above your head, feet together. Swing arms forward, and slowly curl up the upper torso as hands reach toward thighs;

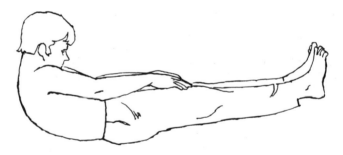

hands should go about halfway down the thighs. Uncurl slowly, and lie down again. Boys: eight times; girls: five times.

WAIST, BACK, INNER THIGHS

Sit on floor with legs apart in wide V. Back straight, arms outstretched straight from the shoulders. Twist to the left while swinging right arm down to touch left toes with fingers.

Keep knees straight. Repeat with left arm. Boys: ten times; girls: six.

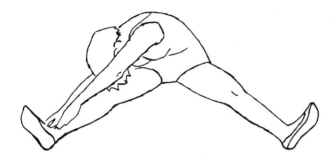

HIPS, OUTER THIGHS

Lie on floor on left side with left arm folded under head and right hand on floor in front of chest for balance. Right leg will be on top of left leg. Slowly lift the right leg, pointing toes, to about eighteen inches above the left one. Hold for count of five, then continue lifting as high as is comfortable.

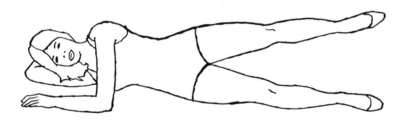

Return downward, repeat hold at same place, and lower leg to original position. Switch position and do it with the other leg. Five times.

HIPS, WAIST, MIDRIFF

Lie on your stomach with elbows bent in front of you. Raise chin up and back, keeping head in straight line (that is, don't *turn* your head). Push upper torso back with arms while bringing feet up as if to meet back of head (you can bend your knees!). Five times, gently.

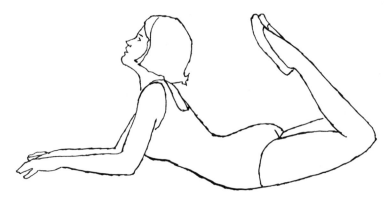

WAIST

Stand erect, feet about a foot and a half apart. Arms out to sides at shoulder level. Twist in a forward swing and touch right toes with left fingers. Return to original position, and repeat with opposite toes/fingers. Boys: ten times each foot; girls: five times each foot. (This should be vigorous and quick.)

THIGHS AND HIPS

Lie on your stomach with elbows slightly bent in front of you. Raise chin up, but keep head level ahead. Bring up right

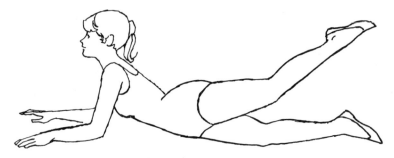

leg and hip, with knee bent, toes pointing to ceiling. This one looks a bit like a backward kick while lying down. But gently does it. Ten times each leg.

HIPS AND THIGHS

Stand erect, feet slightly apart, arms stretched out in front. Rise to tiptoe, then slowly squat down to half sitting position. Return slowly to standing position. Repeat ten times.

For Boys Only

Developing bulging muscles can very often cause the overweight boy to appear even more overweight. Your main concern should be with tightening and strengthening your entire musculature and making it flexible.

Nevertheless, if you want to build big muscles, you can use any of the well-known systems, such as calisthenics and isometrics (never use unless followed immediately with aerobics); or you can get a good program from your gym teacher.

Jogging and swimming both can give you the best physique for your body build without muscle mass.

EXPERIMENT No. 3

This experiment is in two parts, and is to be used with your overall exercise program. You will see it listed on the Exercise Program Chart with minimum performance times each week.

Part One

MINIMUM TIME: 3 minutes

BEST TIME TO PRACTICE: about half an hour before lunch or dinner. (For the sake of discussion, we will assume that your long-range weight loss goal is twenty pounds. Substitute your real goal when you do the experiment.)

Sit quietly for a few moments (alone, if possible) with your eyes closed. Conjure up a mental picture of yourself twenty pounds lighter. "See" in your mind every detail of the picture. Imagine how you feel, what you are wearing, what you're doing. Fix the twenty-pounds-lighter-you firmly in mind.

Now, go back over the steps you will go through to get there. Build a mental scenario of your step-by-step procedure for arriving at your desired weight level. See yourself dieting sensibly and following the Basic Diet Plan; add to the picture your exercise program—how you're doing it day by day.

See yourself arriving at each five-pound target and then going on to the next with the diet/exercise routine each day.

Spend a few minutes rehearsing your mental movie. Telegraph the entire message to the Inner Man. Keep flashing the picture of yourself as very active, following your diet, and losing weight.

Part Two

MINIMUM TIME: 3 minutes

BEST TIME TO PRACTICE: when you first wake up in the morning. (This part of the experiment should be done on *alternate* days.)

Part One concentrates on your overall program. This part brings you to your intermediate targets, one by one.

If your first five-pound loss brings you to, say, 135 pounds, this is the figure you will concentrate on. Your next one will be 130 pounds, and so on.

Close your eyes and visualize clearly in your mind's eye the number 135—just as if it were written in huge numerals on a big piece of cardboard. See it in your mind as sharply as you read it on the bathroom scale.

Then "see" yourself going through the steps to arrive at a five-pound loss, just as you rehearsed your overall program in Part One. You are eating sensibly, watching your diet, and you're exercising. What you're doing is mentally rehearsing this one segment of your program—everything you're doing to lose the five pounds. Do this experiment in turn for each target.

Then, after you have rehearsed the experiment in your mind, take a full-sized sheet of note paper, and write your target in bold letters. Stick the sheet to your bedroom mirror, pin it on the wall, or inside your closet door—anywhere you will see it within a few minutes after you come home. Change the paper and the place you pin it up each time you do the experiment.

YOUR EXERCISE PROGRAM

CATEGORY I: up to 6 pounds overweight

You don't have a weight problem yet—you have a backside problem. You've spent too much time warming the bench. Take the Personal Survey tests of your calorie intake and energy expenditure (pages 94, 96) to see which needs changing. You may be able to cut just the extra Cop-out Calories.

Choose some exercises from the group on page 107, and begin the program for Category II. Concentrate mainly on more activity.

And give yourself a chance; unless both parents are overweight, you probably have no problem except impatience.

CATEGORY II: 6 to 10 pounds overweight

TIME: 3 to 5 weeks

MINIMUM CALORIE INTAKE:

Boys, 15,400 per week, averaging 2,200 a day

Girls, 12,600 per week, averaging 1,800 a day

MAXIMUM CALORIE INTAKE:

Boys, 16,800 per week, averaging 2,400 a day

Girls, 14,000 per week, averaging 2,000 a day

SECOND WEEK:

Look for your First Plateau to appear.

AFTER FIFTH WEEK:

This is the time for averaging out and reassessing your intake-output ratio.

CATEGORY III: 11 to 20 pounds overweight. (You must complete Basic Unit One before you begin.)

MINIMUM CALORIE INTAKE:

You may need to readjust upward. How many pounds have you lost since you began? Divide by five to get your average (you must include the first week, regardless of how big a weight loss you may have had. You should be losing NO MORE than two pounds, no less than one a week.

FIRST ADJUSTMENT:

If you're losing faster, add in Basic Diet Units to bring your food intake back up. Allow 1,700 calories a week for each half-pound adjustment.

If you *aren't* losing at the proper average, re-examine your diet. Are you counting everything you eat? Look for uncounted calories, and check your exercise schedule. Are you giving it a good go or goofing off?

	BASIC UNIT ONE	1st week	2nd week	3rd week	4th week	5th week
EXPERIMENT No. 2	3 min.	daily	every other day	same	same	same
EXPERIMENT No. 3 (Parts 1 & 2)	6 min.	twice weekly	same	same	same	same
AEROBICS Jogging Biking Swimming	30 min. or segments	daily	same add 5 min. (35)	same add 5 min. (40)	same add 5 min. (45)	same same
ADD-ONS Three warm-ups Two flexibility Two figure shapers	15 min.	every other day	same	same	five times a week	five times a week
BOOSTERS	6 kinds	daily	daily	daily	daily	daily

By the end of the fifth week, you should be much more active in general and finding many ways to boost your energy output.

YOUR EXERCISE PROGRAM

CATEGORY IV: Over 20 pounds overweight

REMEMBER:

A medical checkup is a MUST for this category. Get your doctor's okay before you tackle a weight loss program.

COMPLETE BASIC UNITS ONE AND TWO BEFORE BEGINNING THIS UNIT.

MINIMUM CALORIE INTAKE:

How are you averaging? You should settle down to losing a steady one to one and a half pounds a week (although you may not lose *every* week). By now, your average should work out to the above figures.

If not, you're taking in too many calories and not getting enough exercise. Are you weighing your food? Are you measuring it? Are you *really* spending the full time in activity and really putting out the energy?

	BASIC UNIT TWO	6th week	7th week	8th week	9th week	10th week
EXPERIMENT No. 2	3 min.	twice weekly	same	same	same	same
EXPERIMENT No. 3 (Parts 1 & 2)	6 min.	once weekly	same	same	same	same
AEROBICS Jogging Swimming Biking	45 min.	every day	same	add 5 min. (50)	same (50)	add 10 min. (60)
ADD-ONS Three warm-ups Two flexibility Two figure shapers	15 min.	six	six	daily	daily	daily
BOOSTERS	6 kinds	daily	daily	daily	daily	daily

Note: You may expect your Second Plateau somewhere about the ninth week. Don't change your diet. Give your body a chance to coast for a while. After a couple of weeks, increase your energy output.

BASIC UNIT THREE		*11th week*	*12th week*	*13th week*	*14th week*	*15th week*	*16th week, etc.*
EXPERIMENT No. 2	3 min.	twice weekly	same	same	same	same	continuing twice weekly
EXPERIMENT No. 3 (Parts 1 & 2)	6 min.	once weekly	same	same	same	same	continuing once weekly
AEROBICS Jogging Biking Swimming	60 min.	daily	daily	daily	daily	daily	daily
		Begin weekly increase at rate of 15 minutes a day to reach a minimum level of two hours a day					
ADD-ONS Three warm-ups Four flexibility Two optional choices	15 min.	daily	daily	daily	daily	daily	daily
BOOSTERS	6 kinds	daily	daily	daily	daily	daily	daily

By the tenth week, your basic maintenance program should include ONE HOUR of aerobics every day plus a minimum of fifteen minutes of add-ons daily.

You should be in top shape now and tackling many kinds of outside activities to bring your vigorous energy level up to two hours a day. Good aerobics: handball, squash, basketball. Try anything that forces you to spend energy; but remember to keep focused on EXERCISE and NOT ON STANDING AROUND WATCHING.

21

HANDLING THE PITFALLS

Your biggest weight loss normally comes during the first ten days to three weeks. The more fat you have to lose, the more you're likely to lose during this period.

For instance, if you're overfat by thirty pounds, you may drop as much as five or ten pounds. But then you should level off to a steady loss averaging one or two pounds a week.

When this leveling off occurs, you've hit your First Plateau. Many dieters go into an emotional tailspin and blow the whole scene when this happens. Their first reaction to the big loss was a whooping, "Let's go for broke!" They got results FAST. Now they want *more* results FASTER.

They react to the leveling off as if they had walked into a stone wall. They lose patience, forget their goal, and bingo, they're in a booby trap. Result: discouragement and failure.

Don't let your First Plateau throw you. Plan for it. *Look for the leveling off after the big drop to signal your success.* It means you've hit your first target, you're right on course, and all signals are go!

The Second Plateau

There's no way to pinpoint your second leveling off period. Again, it depends upon your weight, growth, and individual body mechanisms. It could happen at six weeks, three months, or six months.

But when it does come, celebrate! It's time for cheers, not tears! You've reached your second big triumph, and now your body is ready for a rest. All that hard, nitty-gritty work it's been doing has paid off, and you've reset your balance at a lower level.

Whatever you do, *don't step up the pressure by cutting calories!* Give your body a chance to coast along for a while and catch its breath; it's earned a break. Continue your program as usual.

After a few weeks, when no further weight loss shows up, you can step up your activity schedule gradually, and you'll begin losing weight again at a steady pace.

Averaging Out

Over the period of your individual program, your weight loss should average *no more* than two pounds a week. Category IV people may average two pounds a week until they get down to Category III; then the weight loss should taper down to one and a half pounds.

Note the key word: average. This means that your loss will vary from week to week. The first week or so your loss will be highest; and during your plateau weeks, you may not lose anything. The key to performance is the long-range averaging.

If you find yourself losing too fast, you must add back Food Units: 1,700 calories in extra food per week for each half pound you're losing too fast.

If you aren't averaging a minimum of one pound a week, your activity level is much too low; step it up in all departments.

Handling the Temptations

The inevitable day of irresistible temptation will arrive. This is the day you can't resist the calorie-laden Cop-outs. The day has come for blowing the diet sky-high.

Don't sweat it. Blow the diet if you must. *Just keep your long-range goal in mind at all times,* and you'll find your temptation days getting fewer and farther between.

You can work off the extra calories by adding in a few additional minutes of exercise for the next week or so.

Remember, you're only human—don't try to be an angel twenty-four hours a day!

22

TAKING EMOTIONAL STOCK

Some teen-agers will need to think twice about their emotional readiness for a weight loss program. Ask yourself some straightforward questions, and give honest answers.

Except for your overweight (which is enough of a problem), is the rest of your scene in fairly even balance? Or are you in the middle of turmoil? If there is serious trouble in your life—for instance, a deep unhappiness over other problems—you may have enough to handle.

Some people find in a big emotional problem just the spur they need to motivate them to change their lives. You may be one of these people; you may not. Weigh your present emotional climate realistically. *Then* decide if you're really ready to tackle the weight loss program.

If you have any doubts about your emotional readiness, wait a while before you start the diet. Instead, begin the exercise program, and follow through with it. When you feel more secure and self-confident about things, you can start your calorie controls.

Remember that most weight loss programs that depend only on calorie controls are rough. The pressures inside and out are enormous, and frequent depressions result. That's one major reason for balancing diet with exercise.

Exercise is your safety valve for letting off emotional steam and easing the stresses. *Never try any diet control scheme without a parallel exercise program*—and DON'T pick up only the diet part of this one either!

Taking Your Temperature

All through your program, you must take your emotional temperature. Learn to recognize the moods that warn you of when the pressure is building.

Depressions can be a danger signal. It's time for *action!* It's time to change your routine—get out, do things, be with people, keep yourself too busy to think about your problems. One hour—repeat: ONE HOUR—is the TOP TIME LIMIT for a depressed mood! Never give it a chance to grab you. Drop everything, and do something silly, wild, and fun, even if it means blowing your diet for the day. You can pick it right up again with a simple input/output adjustment the next morning, and you're still on course.

Irritability may be another danger signal. (It *may* be. Like the guy wearing a hair shirt, you could have good reason to itch.) But general irritability and unhappiness without apparent cause can signal the need for a change of activities and routine. You may need some spice in your life. You're in a rut and chafing; get out and mix with people. It's time to circulate more, subordinate your problems to those of groups or individuals working for some of the long-range goals that will make our world a better place for living.

The longer you're in your program, the more sensitive you will become to the wiles and strategies of the detractors. It's perfectly normal to react with impatience to those who have little insight or understanding. In fact, it can be a healthy, self-protective reaction. If you have valid reason to blow your stack, do it. Never be afraid to stick up for yourself when someone shortchanges you. On the other hand, never be afraid to give or accept an apology—or you *could* miss some of the best moments of your life.

Recognize that you will have disappointments, big and little. It's par for the course. Just keep tabs on yourself, and don't blow things up out of proportion, or they'll blow you off your course. You have time on your side—time to change the disappointments into triumphs. So get to work, and slice them down to bite size.

YOUR BEST FOOT FORWARD

You're losing weight because you want to look better. So here are a few simple guidelines to help you look your best.

Your Complexion

There's no big mystique about skin care, in spite of the outlandish claims of advertisers. A clear, radiant skin is a reflection of good health, simple cleanliness, and the "you" behind the face.

But there *is* a "skin problem" stage that's quite common among teen-agers. You know the name of that stage well. It's called "acne" by doctors. Acne is the technical term for a lot of plaguing pimples.

Acne has nothing to do with morals or manners. It isn't a result of any behavior on your part. What actually causes it is not clearly understood, but dermatologists (skin specialists) believe it is triggered by the speedup in hormone secretions during adolescence.

There's no "cure" for it, and it can't be prevented. It *will* respond to treatment in many cases.

A diet that emphasizes vegetables and fruits and de-emphasizes sweets and fats is frequently recommended by specialists. Careful attention to cleanliness also helps until the skin adjusts to hormonal changes.

Usually, warm water and ordinary soap are sufficient cleansers for the average person. Cleanliness—especially that of the hands and scalp—is one of the most important preventive methods.

Indiscriminate use of "cure" cosmetics may irritate an already sensitive skin. The specialists feel that each case of acne is highly individual and no one product or method is necessarily effective for everyone. What works for you might irritate someone else's skin.

A minimum amount of care consists of washing your face with warm water and mild soap or detergent in the morning and again at night. If your skin is very oily (it gets shiny within a couple of hours after washing), or if you're in a period of skin eruptions, you may need to wash your face more often.

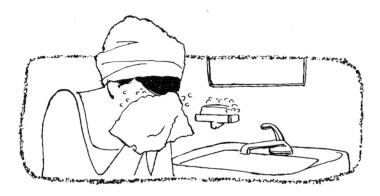

A mild soap acts as a drying agent, removing the upper layer of dead skin cells and unplugging the pores. The hard, dried oil that plugs skin pores at the surface is responsible for the beginnings of pimples. When the hardened oil oxidizes, it turns dark, and we call the plugged pore a blackhead.

Don't squeeze pimples. It's hard to resist, but you actually cause greater damage. Squeezing breaks down the tissues around the pimple and causes scarring. It isn't something you will notice immediately. It's cumulative over a period of time. You also run the risk of greater infection, particularly around the nose and mouth area.

If you have a severe problem, or if the acne doesn't subside within a few months, see your dermatologist. *Girls:* Discontinue make-up when you're plagued with skin eruptions. Wait until they recede before you resume use of make-up. The hypo-allergenic cosmetics won't necessarily help since the idea is to keep the skin pores free of anything that will clog them.

Your Hair

If you have acne problems, you probably have scalp problems, too. They usually go together. A severe case of dandruff is thought to be caused by glands also.

Avoid self-treatment with salves, lotions, and whatnot. A gentle shampoo with plenty of warm water can usually help most. Wash your hair as frequently as needed, not on any sort of Monday and Thursday schedule. Rinse well.

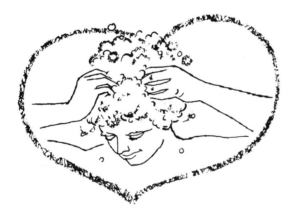

Stay away from bleaches, dyes, tints, and anything caustic until the problem is solved. You may irritate or damage scalp tissue permanently. Brush your hair thoroughly every day to loosen and brush out the loose skin scales.

It is very important to keep the hair scrupulously clean and off the face when you have acne. Hair blowing or falling on the face aggravates the acne and may cause it to spread.

Simple dandruff, which is just a normal shedding of the dry upper skin layers (unsightly, but not serious), can be controlled by daily brushing and shampooing when needed.

Sun and sea will dry both hair and skin, so take a little extra care during the summer. Always shower (hair, too, if it gets wet) after swimming. Use a light oil or lotion on the body to replace lost lubricants (baby oil is great). Dry hair will usually respond to light touchups with hair-conditioning ointments.

Dry-skin problems after shower or bath may be due to hard water or to a slight allergic reaction to the soap you're using. Try changing soaps or using a water softener in the bath. In the shower, use a soap with built-in softener. Use light oil as body lotion immediately after showering.

Dress for De-emphasis

The more overweight you are, the more attention you must give to your appearance. Neatness and cleanliness are very important assets for you.

Neatness is mostly careful attention to details of dress. Are clothes clean and pressed? No missing buttons? No sagging hems? Hair neat and well-groomed? Hands clean, and fingernails trimmed and clean? No runs in stockings or pantyhose, if you wear them? No food stains down the shirt front? The most smashing costume you can wear will be utterly ruined by one hanging thread or popped seam simply because these things are so noticeable!

Styles in clothes change rapidly, and personal preferences vary widely. But any style should "hang together" or have a look of being complete and harmonious. And clothes should be right for the occasion. No party velveteens at a football game, for instance.

You can improve your general appearance tremendously by observing a few general tips:

—Avoid extreme styles in clothes.
Understatement should be your keynote.

—Girls: stay away from busy frills, gathered or heavily pleated skirts, dresses with gobs of material, tight body shirts, and materials that cling to every curve. They really don't disguise anything, and they do call more attention to your extra pounds.

—Avoid clothes with big, bold designs such as large plaids, stripes (particularly horizontal), geometrics, florals. Nothing big and busy helps at all.

—Best bets are outfits of one color or one design. If you choose separates, they should match or blend. Avoid anything in style or color that chops you in half horizontally.

—Choose smooth, nonbulky fabrics. Avoid tweeds and heavy woolens.

—Dark colors usually tend to de-emphasize your overweight. But don't avoid the bright colors. Just keep your costume all of one solid color.

—(Sometimes you need a bright color to zing you up and brighten your mood. So go right ahead and wear that bright red or green whenever you need a cheerful lift!)

—Unless you're quite good (and tasteful!) at it, don't mix designs—even the small ones you'll be wearing. Simplicity should be your keynote in dress; no fuss, frills, or anything overstated. You'll have plenty of chance to get flamboyant when you lose the excess weight!

—Avoid large, chunky jewelry, especially chokers or necklaces. If your hands are too chubby (many overweights don't gain in their hands, curiously enough), don't wear large or flashy rings.

—Buying something new? When you're ready, be sure to try it on first. Look at yourself in a three-way mirror so you can really see if it fits correctly and if it does something for you.

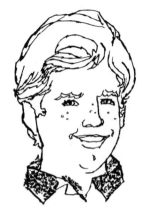

Hair Styles

The long-haired styles so popular now aren't the greatest "look" for the overweight guy or gal. Generally, the best hair styles are the in-between ones for the guys. The simple, shorter ones are best for girls. But if you prefer long hair, keep it under control with barrettes, bobby pins, a pony tail, or in the way you have it styled and cut.

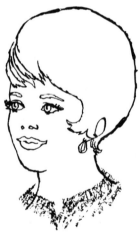

Make-up

Your keynote in make-up is the natural look. Accentuate your good points with restraint, and de-emphasize bad points.

Tone down cheeks with a dark toner or darker shade of face powder. Use dark toner under the chin to de-emphasize a too-fat chin. Go easy on the eye make-up—remember that nobody was ever born with blue, green, or silver eyelids. Save the eye shadows for evening, and then be sure you use them as subtle accents.

Firm-ups for Flabby Face and Neck Muscles

Add into your regular exercise program these special muscle toners for the face and neck. They will help tighten and trim you faster.

CHIN AND NECK SLIMMER

Lie down across your bed on your back. Let your head hang well down over the side of the bed. Slowly bring your head up until it is level with your body. Hold for a slow count of five. Then bring your head up as close as possible to your chest. Hold for another slow five. Lower the head back down, very s-l-o-w-l-y. Girls: three times; boys: six times.

CHIN AND NECK SLIMMER

Sit tall and straight on edge of bed, with head high, neck raised from your shoulders. Lower your head backwards very slowly as far as possible. Now open your mouth as wide as possible, keeping head in back position. Close mouth, bringing bottom lip up over top lip. Hold for a slow five count. Repeat five times.

THE SWING AROUND

Sit tall as before. Drop chin to chest, and begin slow head roll, rotating the head toward the right shoulders, on to the back, dropping head far back, on to the left shoulder, and return chin to chest position. Repeat three times in both directions.

24

MAKING YOUR WAVES

Spotting the Detractors

Few people understand the problems of the overweight. Even fewer understand the problems of losing weight. On your way down, you will meet the same devil's disciples you met on your way up. The trick is to spot them and learn to deal with them.

A real pal will be sympathetic and cheer you on. This is the angel who's been in your corner all along.

Recognize that about 99 percent of the people around you think you are overweight because you lack the "will power" to stop overeating. Actually, there's no such thing as "will power." It's simply a catchall label to explain behavior one doesn't understand. There is always a reason, or a complex set of reasons, why we do something or don't do it.

As you've learned, the overweight must deal with a combination of physical, mental, and social pressures. Understanding some of the social pressures can give you insight to help you cope with your problems.

Pay no attention to people who tell you that you're looking drawn and haggard—it's all in their minds. They need time to get accustomed to the new you, to "seeing" you differently.

Tell them you're losing weight sensibly and slowly. Even a small weight loss often shows first in your face. It will take a little time while your body readjusts. Meanwhile, chalk one up for you—you're making waves.

People who persist in criticizing are really trying to undermine your program. Be firm and blunt. Tell them they will get used to it! But know them for what they are—the same characters who react negatively when you *gain* weight!

When you undertake a weight loss program, you create subtle changes in the world around you. Everyone will react to your new "role." Some will find it confusing and vaguely threatening because you're stepping out of character. Others will be envious of your new-found "will power" (as they see it).

Another tough nut to handle is the one who tries to get you off your diet. He will urge all sorts of temptations on the theory that it won't hurt "just this once." The world of the dieter is full of "onces" that add up to a blown diet. Resist; essentially, it's the other person's problem, not yours. What he really wants is company. He's dying to indulge himself in that luscious strawberry sundae. When you firmly resist it, *he* feels guilty if he indulges!

Of course, there's always Mr. Ridicule. But you've met him before. He operates the same way in every department by putting other people down. Learn to ignore him. He's really a bully. When you don't react to his ridicule, he will tire quickly and look around for another scapegoat. He has to; it's the only way he knows to handle his problems.

Handling the Dinner Party

It isn't necessary to discuss your diet unless you want to. Your best bet is to eat a small portion of everything and to compliment your hostess. There's no rule requiring you to finish your plate or to take second helpings.

The hostess who insists on overfeeding you is like the hostess who insists on serving a cocktail to a guest who doesn't drink. In either case, her bad manners are showing, and she needs firm handling.

Many people are impatient with dieters and seem to regard the whole thing as a lark not to be taken seriously. At best, their attitude is one of indifference. But you can't change people unless you educate them. And education isn't your goal, weight control is.

It won't be long before you can spot the detractors a block away. You'll learn to anticipate them and to deal with them. Speak up for yourself, and let the other guy know that *his* attitudes are *his* problem, not yours. You are, after all, *handling* yours.

How Did You Get That Cheering Section?

Very simple. Time did it for you. After everyone gets adjusted to the new routine, they come over to your side, one by one.

This is where you pull out that sense of humor! Expect your cheering section to get into the act with you. Your program becomes theirs, and before you know it, they will keep score right along with you.

Keep your cool. Don't get aggravated when they count your calories, watch your diet, tell you what's "fattening" and what isn't, and want to come jogging with you.

Just remember, it's *their* way of cheering you on. The more involved they get in your routine, the more they care about what you're doing. It's proof you've made your waves and you're changing your world.

There's only one solution: grin and bear it. And congratulate yourself!

25

JUST FOR MOM

You're the most important ingredient, Mom. Your understanding and cooperation are essential to your teen-ager's success in losing weight—and *keeping it off*.

You'll wear several hats. The most important one is that of cheerleader, because your attitudes and actions will help set the tone for the rest of the family. You can make the job of losing weight a more positive, less painful experience. Losing weight is never easy, but *it can be done*—with your help.

If your teen-ager has been persistently and visibly overweight for long, he is doubly vulnerable to the normal confusions and conflicts that go with the transition to adulthood. Growing up is difficult enough, but growing up overweight can be a shattering experience.

As nutrition expert Dr. Jean Mayer says, ". . . the obese young people in the United States are under constant pressure to become something they are not, and to think poorly of themselves as they are."

When the overweight teen-ager diets and fails, he alone is blamed for his "sin." He alone suffers the pressures, discriminations, and censorious attitudes leveled against him for his "lack of will power." The resulting sense of guilt and rejection can plunge him deeper into social isolation, emotional passivity, and withdrawal from the kinds of outside activities that offer opportunity for exercise.

How Can You Help?

If your overweight teen-ager is *overeating,* take an honest look at yourself and your family to see if you are unwittingly contributing to the problem. Are you from the "eat-eat-they're-starving-in-India" school? Do you insist that family members clean their plates or have second helpings, whether they want them or not?

Or do you serve outsized portions to begin with? Are your menus heavily laden with fats and carbohydrates in the form of rich desserts, breads, gravies, pastas, fried foods?

Is food used as reward, bribe, or punishment? For instance, did the "good boy" get a piece of candy, and was the "bad boy" sent to bed without supper?

Eating habits and food choices are learned early and are *very* hard to break. Using food as a way of giving or withholding approval creates emotional feelings toward food that are quite unconnected with nutritional needs or with actual hunger. Overeating may become the only way a child can deal with situations of stress; or it may be his way of winning approval and reassurance. For a child who is susceptible to overweight, growing up may mean entering a lifelong struggle with excess pounds.

If your overweight teen-ager isn't overeating but *is* underactive, help him to figure out ways to change faulty eating habits and food choices. Very often, many calories can be cut simply by selecting different kinds of foods. The important thing is that he learns to choose nutritious foods.

Encouraging the underactive teen-ager to get moving for the first time can be a difficult job. It's really a new way of life quite different from the cocoon of inactivity to which he's accustomed. Once he makes that first shift into high gear, he finds out that he's having fun. Then his own natural enthusiasm will take over.

Very often, the teen-ager's attitude toward exercise is an echo of the family's. How about the family's general activity level? Does exercise get the spotlight or the brush-off? If the answer is "brush-off," chances are there are other family members who have a weight problem also! Perhaps you can get everyone to begin an exercise program—for weight control as well as good health.

(Out-of-condition adults shouldn't tackle the teen-agers' jogging program, however. Give yourself ten to sixteen weeks to work up to a continuous daily jog of thirty minutes; the other exercises can be taken in stride for any normally healthy adult.)

Watching Those Calories

There are a number of great low-calorie cookbooks in inexpensive paperback form on the market. And hundreds of recipes are published in the monthly magazines every year. In fact, so much calorie information has been published that you can figure the count of almost any food eaten by the average American family.

Why not start your own collection of recipes and cooking tips now? Enlist the aid of your overweight teen-ager as well as the help of other family members. You'll find that food choices are enormous, and dieting need not be so difficult after all. Using the Basic Unit plan, your overweight teen-ager can (usually) have the same menu as the rest of the family, just less of it.

Counting calories in your cooking isn't difficult. A good program for a rainy afternoon is to go through your recipe file with the calorie counter handy. Write in your recipe book the calorie counts of ingredients; each time you copy a recipe, make a note of the calories and how much a serving equals. (See page 139 for directions in figuring recipes.)

Suppose, for instance, that you wanted to serve a potato salad. You could figure the ingredients and find out that one serving would be approximately eighty calories. Looking under the Basic Foods Units, you see that white potatoes are listed as a Breads/Cereals. So, the potato salad would be your teen-ager's Breads/Cereals Unit, with one Fats Unit for the mayonnaise.

You can save thousands of calories a year with a little

extra attention to cooking and food preparation before cooking. Buy the leanest cuts of meats, and trim all visible fats. Omit, or cut drastically, the fats and oils called for in many standard recipes.

For instance, the sautéing step can frequently be eliminated, particularly in stews and sauces that must cook for a while. You can also sauté using bouillon, or meat drippings with added water (fat well-drained, please!), or by oven braising roasts or other meats you usually sear in fat.

Broil, bake, or roast meats on racks so that fats drain off. Restrict fried and breaded dishes to a minimum since they do add lots of extra calories.

Teflon pans are the greatest inventions yet for cutting the fat calories. Try them for both meats and vegetables. Replace the traditional butter in vegetable cookery with a small piece of very lean ham or Canadian bacon. Save vegetable juices for between-meal snacks.

Close attention to nutritional balance will frequently take care of the calories. Balancing a starchy vegetable with a leafy green, for instance, will average out in calories.

Slow down pesky appetites with low-calorie appetizers: a slice of melon, cup of broth or soup (nonfatty) before dinner. Cut calories in creamed soup by substituting skimmed milk or water for whole milk, and serve soup in half-cup portions.

Be generous with tossed salads at any meal, and serve them as the first course. Just remember to count the dressing as a Fats Unit.

Serve fish often—it's a great source of top-quality protein and is generally lower in calories than meat. Just cook without adding in calories from sauces.

Sharing the Kitchen

Don't make your teen-ager feel that the kitchen is off-limits. Learning about foods, about caloric and nutritional values, about food preparation and how to cut calories, is invaluable training. Your teen-ager's weight problem will not disappear, or be "cured," when he loses the excess pounds. He will be susceptible to overweight the minute he reverts to his old way of life. What he learns now about good nutrition and balanced diet will serve him well in later years when his activity level gradually decreases.

An interest in learning about foods will help also to keep him on his course and will make him constantly alert to his eating habits. Knowing the caloric and nutritional values of foods shows him how to make better choices to meet both requirements.

If your teen-ager hasn't worked in the kitchen before, sit down with him or her and draw up some basic ground rules for use of the kitchen. A few moments of your time explaining correct (and safe!) use of gadgets can save many arguments later.

If necessary, set up fair and square rules for cleaning up and putting things away.

Let your teen-ager help in planning the food buying. Together you may figure out numerous ways to save calories without penalizing the appetite or the family.

Try to keep temptation to an absolute minimum, especially during the first few weeks of dieting or during a slump. Keep on hand plenty of low-calorie, nutritious foods for snacking. Be sure they are well separated from high-calorie nibbles and kept in a convenient spot.

If the rest of the family (the nonoverweight ones) must have their candy, cakes, and potato chips, store them out of sight. Urge other family members to have snacks when your dieter isn't around. Don't put undue or unfair stress on your teen-ager's appetite controls. Remember that normal-weight people frequently expect impossible restraint on the part of a dieter.

How to Calculate Calories in a Recipe and Figure Out an Individual Serving

Write down the individual ingredients and their amounts. Look up the number of calories in each item, and calculate them according to the amounts called for in the recipe. (The endpapers in this book show you measurements by weight and by volume.) Add total number of calories and divide by the number of servings in recipe to get calories for one serving.

26

YOUR MONEY'S WORTH

Every year, fakes and swindlers bilk the American public of over one billion dollars. According to the Post Office, reducing schemes alone skim off a whopping $100 million. Unnecessary or falsely represented vitamin products and "health" foods grab another $500 million.

Hundreds of nonprescription pills and props are available to the unwary in drugstores, supermarkets, and department stores all over the country. Every newspaper and magazine carries at least one ad for some sure-fire "miracle diet," gadget, or what have you.

None of these schemes or products can do a thing for you that you can't do for yourself with *no investment*.

This isn't to put down the exercise gadgets. Some of them are effective. But so are your own exercises at home without the expense.

There's really only one known prop that can control your weight—it's called *motivation*. It's more effective than any pill or scheme you can buy.

While We're on the Subject

Amphetamines are prescription drugs that have been widely used as appetite depressants in treating the overweight. Many doctors prescribe them at the beginning of a diet in order to get the patient going. But they have been "oversold" as a cure for overweight. They are nothing more than a temporary stopgap. In the long run, they don't belong in any intelligent weight loss program. Why?

Using these drugs is a little like taking an aspirin for a headache. You're relieving the *symptom* for the moment but doing nothing about the *cause*. Eventually, you must come to grips with your problem in terms of changing your eating patterns and your activity levels.

The amphetamines are usually effective for only about six weeks, so you're back where you started: facing the basic problem. Meanwhile, you've lost the six weeks with a prop that's taken the initiative away from you.

But the kicker in a pill program is this—when the program fails, the victim gets the blame. But the pill gets the credit for dazzling "results" (after all, you *did* lose the weight; it's your own fault if you gained it back).

Foods, Fads, Facts

"Health foods" are no different from ordinary foods. They just cost a lot more. With the extra cost comes the health foods mystique, a strange blend of pseudo-scientific "nutrition" and plain old-fashioned bunk.

Four major myths pop up over and over. These are:

Myth 1: Our "impoverished" soils produce nutritionally deficient foods.

TRUTH: American soil is the world's richest, and it's the farmer's most precious asset. You can bet he takes good care of it. Poor soil produces a poor yield and smaller plants, but studies have proved there's no measurable nutritional deficiency. Nutritious foods come from the kinds of *seeds* planted more than the kind of soil. The statement is absurd on the face of it—the yield per acre of American soil is so high that we *pay* farmers not to produce!

Myth 2: Organically grown foods are more nutritious and retain their natural flavor.

TRUTH: Nutritionally, there's no difference. The "organic" claque claims that chemical fertilizers ruin and devitalize crops. It simply isn't so. If a plant needs nitrogen (a

141

chemical!), for instance, it will convert it from whatever source. It's still nitrogen. The "organic" fertilizers help to produce a loamier soil that makes it easier for young plants to take root.

Food flavor depends upon when the food is gathered, how soon it reaches the market, and how long it stays on the shelf or counter before you buy it.

Myth 3: Processing devitalizes food.

TRUTH: Complete nonsense. Modern methods of food processing help preserve nutritional values. Quick-frozen fruits and vegetables, for instance, are more likely to retain their nutritional values than are fresh foods. Why? Because they are processed immediately after picking and before they lose their flavor and nutrients through oxidation and dehydration.

Myth 4: Americans suffer from vitamin and mineral deficiencies caused by poor food. Therefore, they should eat the "health foods."

TRUTH: Some Americans *do* have vitamin or mineral deficiencies. Many teenagers' diets are frequently low in iron and calcium. But this isn't due to devitalized foods—it's due to an imbalanced diet. Teen-agers don't eat enough proteins, milk, and leafy vegetables, even when their families can well afford to buy them. A well-balanced diet of ordinary foods from the supermarket will provide you with vitamins and minerals, and at much less cost than the health foods.

Many of the food faddists are quite sincere in their beliefs about the miracles of health foods. They will tell you glowing stories of "cures" for all types of ailments, most of which are self-diagnosed. They vow they "never felt better" in their lives.

The truth is that they are giving more time and attention to what they eat. Consequently, they are more likely to get a better-balanced diet. Who wouldn't feel better?

Health foods are not harmful. The harm lies in the mistaken belief in their miraculous powers of "curing" all manner of ailments. Many people incorrectly diagnose their own ailments and fail to seek medical help because of their faith in health food "cures."

Magic Foods?

Some of the most common "miracle" foods are:

YOGURT: It's a milk product and has the same kinds of nutrients. No magic powers for reducing either. It has approximately 160 calories per cup (depending on the brand).

BLACKSTRAP MOLASSES: Claimed to be a rich source of iron. But you get more iron, of better quality, from liver, oysters, pork, organ meats, dried beans/peas, and dark green leafy vegetables. The so-called "minerals" in blackstrap molasses are mainly the impurities that result from the refining process.

KELP (SEAWEED): Supposedly for your iodine deficiency. Normal use of ordinary iodized table salt, or frequent seafoods on your menu, will give you all you need.

HONEY: An excellent food and a good replacement for sugar since you get some nutrients without too many additional calories. But there's nothing magic enough to justify paying 50–100 per cent more for it in a health food shop!

The same holds true for many foods, such as unflavored gelatin and wheat germ. These are two really fine foods that should be used generously in your diet, but they have no "magic" other than the same wholesomeness that other nutritious foods have.

If your health is precarious enough to require such "special" magic, then you need medical attention.

CALORIE CHART

PROTEIN ITEMS

(* indicates one Basic Protein Unit)

	Average Calories		Average Calories
American cheese, 4 slices	210 *	Corned beef hash, 6 oz.	240 *
Bacon, Canadian-style, crisp, drained, 5 slices	250 *	Cottage cheese, ¾ cup	162 *
		Crab meat, canned/ cooked, 1 cup	168 *
Beans, peas, dried, cooked, ¾ cup	230 *	Eggs, 2, cooked without butter	154 *
Beef, 3 ounces, lean, all visible fat removed	245 *	Fish, 4 ounces, fresh, frozen (baked or broiled only)	192 *
Black-eyed peas, ½ cup	100		
Cheddar and other hard cheeses, 2 ounces	210 *	Frogs' legs, fried, 3 large	213 *
Chicken, 3 ounces, lean, roasted, baked, stewed	256 *	Gelatin, plain, dry, 1 tbsp.	34
		Kidney beans, canned, 1 cup	240 *
Chicken, Southern-fried, ½ breast, or 2 medium legs, or 1 leg, 1 thigh	232 *	Lamb, lean, all visible fat removed, 3 ounces	258 *
Chicken, baked, roasted, stewed, 1 small breast, or ¼ small broiler	200 *	Lobster, canned/fresh, 1 cup	160 *
		Lobster, 1 broiled (1½ lbs.)	216 *
Chipped beef, dried, ⅔ cup	224 *	Mozzarella cheese, 2 oz.	220 *
		Oysters, fried, 3 large	204
Clams, raw, ½ doz. medium	86	Oysters, raw, 1½ dozen	225 *
Clams, fried, 10 medium	250 *	Pork, 3 ounces, lean, all visible fat removed	240 *
Codfish cake, 1 large	215 *	Pork, 2 links (3" x ½") or 1 sausage patty, cooked and well drained	250 *
Corned beef, canned, 3 oz.	220 *		

	Average Calories
Pork and beans with tomato sauce, canned, ¾ cup	222 *
With molasses, ¾ cup	243 *
Ricotta cheese, made with partially skimmed milk, ¾ cup	198 *
1 tbsp.	16
With whole milk ½ cup	180 *
1 tbsp.	22½
Salmon, canned, ¾ cup	168 *
Sardines, 1 can (3¾ oz. size), drained	190 *

	Average Calories
Scallops, fried, 3	213 *
Shrimp, canned/fresh, 1 dozen small	64
1 dozen medium	90
Swiss cheese, 2 oz., or about 2 slices	210 *
Tuna, water- or oil-packed, drained, ¾ cup	240 *
Turkey, 3 ounces, any lean portions (including pressed turkey and turkey roll)	228 *
Veal, 3 ounces, lean, all visible fat removed	195 *

FATS ITEMS
(* indicates one Fats Unit)

	Average Calories
Avocado, ½" cubes, or ⅛ cup	45 *
Bacon, crisp, well drained, 1 slice	50 *
Bacon fat, 1 tsp.	42 *
Butter, 1 tsp.	35 *
Chicken fat, 1 tsp.	42 *
Coconut, shredded, 1 tbsp.	42 *
Cream light (sweet or sour), 2 tbsp.	60 *
heavy (sweet), 1 tbsp.	50 *
whipped, 1 heaping tbsp.	50 *
Cream cheese, 1 tbsp.	55 *
Gravy, 1 tbsp.	80 *
Lard, 1 tsp. (pure)	42 *

	Average Calories
Margarine, 1 tsp.	35 *
Mayonnaise, 1 tsp.	35 *
Nuts, 6 small (pecans, filberts, walnuts, almonds, peanuts, etc.)	45 *
Nuts, 2 brazil	56 *
Olives, 6 small, plain, green or black	40
Olives, 3 large, plain, green or black	36 *
Olive oil, 1 tsp.	41 *
Pumpkin seeds, 1 tbsp.	60 *
Peanut butter, 2 tsp.	60 *
Salad dressing, 1 tsp.	35 *
Shortening, 1 tsp.	37 *
Sunflower seeds, shelled, 1 tbsp.	45 *
Vegetable oil, 1 tsp.	42 *

BREADS / CEREALS ITEMS

(* indicates one Basic Breads / Cereals Unit)

	Average Calories		Average Calories
Bagel, ½	60 *	Cheese pastry, Danish, ¼ piece	56 *
Beans, lima, fresh or frozen, ½ cup	75 *	Corn, canned, ½ cup	70 *
Biscuit, ½ small	45 *	Corn, sweet, fresh or frozen, ½ cup or 1 medium cob	85 *
Bran, ¼ cup	47		
Bread		Cornstarch pudding, ¼ cup	70 *
Boston brown, ½ slice	52 *		
raisin, plain, ½ slice	50 *	Crackers, 2 graham	55 *
Thomas' gluten, 1 slice	35 *	4 saltines	50 *
Thomas' protein, 1 slice	45 *	Custard, baked/boiled, ¼ cup	70 *
Rye, whole wheat, white (enriched), 1 slice	60 *	Muffin, ½ English	40 *
Bread crumbs, ⅛ cup	45 *	Noodles, plain, ½ cup	70 *
Breadstick, 1	39 *	Oysterettes (20), ½ cup	60 *
Bun, hamburger or hot dog, ½	60 *	Parsnips, ½ cup	48 *
		Pancake, 1 small	65 *
Cereals, cooked, ½ cup (corn meal mush, farina, grits, oats, oatmeal, cream of rice, rolled whole wheat)	70 *	Potato, 1 small white, baked, with skin, or ½ cup mashed	70 *
		Pretzel stick, 1 small	4
		Rice, cooked, ⅓ cup	60 *
Cereals, unsweetened, ready-to-eat, ¾ cup (corn flakes, oat flakes, puffed rice, Wheaties, etc.)	60 *	Shedded wheat biscuit, ½	45 *
		Spaghetti, cooked, ⅓ cup	56 *
		Toast, melba, plain, 3 slices	60 *
		Zwieback, 1	75 *

147

FRUIT ITEMS

(all items are one Basic Fruits Unit)

	Average Calories		Average Calories
Apple, 1 small	70	Guava, 1 small	49
Apple juice, fresh or canned, ½ cup	62	Honeydew, 2″ x 7″ wedge	49
		Lemons, 2 medium	40
Applesauce, unsweetened, ½ cup	50	Lime, 1½ large	52
Apricots, fresh, 2 medium	51	Loganberries, fresh, ½ cup	45
Apricot halves, dried, 4	60	Mango, 1 small	65
Apricot halves, canned, 3 medium	75	Nectarines, 2 medium	60
		Orange, 1 medium	70
Banana, ½ medium	60	Orange juice, fresh, frozen, canned, ½ cup	55
Blackberries, fresh, ½ cup	40	Papaya, ½ small	45
Blackberries, canned, ¼ cup	54	Peach, fresh, 1 medium	45
		Peaches, frozen, 2 oz.	44
Blueberries, fresh, ½ cup	42	Peach halves, canned, 2	60
Blueberries, frozen, 3 oz. (unsweetened)	52	Pear, 1 small	50
		or 2 halves, canned	50
Blueberries, canned, ¼ cup	60	Pineapple, fresh, ¾ cup	56
Canteloupe, ½, about 5″ in diameter	40	Pineapple, canned, 1 slice	65
Cherries, fresh, 12 large	48	Pineapple juice, fresh, frozen, canned, ½ cup	60
Cherries, canned, ½ cup	61	Plums, fresh, canned, dried, 2 medium	50
Dates, 2 pitted	70	Prunes, uncooked, 2 large	54
Figs, fresh, 2 small	60	Prune juice, ¼ cup	42
Fig, dried, 1 large	55	Raisins, 2 tablespoons	54
Fruit cocktail, canned, ½ cup	45	Raspberries, black, fresh, ½ cup	50
Grapefruit, ½ small	70	Raspberries, red, fresh, ½ cup	35
Grapefruit juice, fresh, frozen, canned, ½ cup	44	Raspberries, red, frozen, 2 oz.	52
Grapes, ½ cup (20)	42	Strawberries, fresh, 1 cup	54
Grape juice, ¼ cup	56	Strawberries, frozen, 1½ oz.	45

	Average Calories		Average Calories
Tangerine, 1 large	45	Watermelon, cubed, 1 cup	56
Tangerine juice, fresh, frozen, canned, ½ cup	45	Watermelon wedge, about ½" x 1" x 10"	55

VEGETABLE ITEMS
(* indicates Basic Vegetable Units)

	Average Calories		Average Calories
Beans, green, cooked, 1 cup	27 *	Mushrooms, fresh, 4 large	16 *
Beet greens, 1 cup	39 *	Mushrooms, canned, 1 cup	30 *
Beets, cooked, ½ cup	35 *	Mustard greens, cooked, 1 cup	31 *
Broccoli, 1 cup	44 *	Okra, cooked, 8 pods	30 *
Brussels sprouts, 1 cup	30 *	Onion, raw, 1 medium	50 *
Cabbage, raw, 1 cup	24 *	Peas, green, ½ cup	56 *
Cabbage, cooked, 1 cup	40 *	Pepper, green, raw, 1 medium	16 *
Cabbage, Chinese, cooked, 1 cup	25 *	Pimientos, canned, 2 medium	20 *
Carrots, cooked, 1 cup	44 *	Pumpkin, canned, ½ cup	38 *
Carrots, raw, 2 medium	42 *	Radishes, 1 medium	5
Cauliflower, raw, 1 cup	25 *	Rutabagas, cooked, ½ cup (yellow turnips)	30 *
Cauliflower, cooked, 1 cup	30 *	Sauerkraut, canned, 1 cup	32 *
Celery, 1 stalk	4	Spinach, cooked, 1 cup	46 *
Chard, 1 cup	30 *	Squash, winter, ½ cup	45 *
Collards, ¾ cup	60 *	Squash, summer, cooked, 1 cup	35 *
Cucumber, raw, 1	25 *	Tomato, fresh, 1 medium	30 *
Dandelion greens, cooked, ½ cup	40 *	Tomato, canned or fresh-cooked, 1 cup	46 *
Eggplant, ½" x 5" slice	20	Tomato juice, 1 cup	50 *
Endive, fresh, 2 stalks	25	Turnips, cooked, 1 cup	42 *
Escarole, fresh, 4 leaves	20	Turnip greens, cooked, 1 cup	43 *
Kale, cooked, 1 cup	44 *	Watercress, fresh, 1 bunch	20
Kohlrabi, fresh, 1 cup	40 *		
Kohlrabi, cooked, 1 cup	47 *		
Lettuce, 1 leaf	3		

SOUP ITEMS
(all are Basic Soup Units)

	Average Calories		Average Calories
Bean soup, ½ cup	50	Madrilene, clear, ½ cup	20
Bouillon (beef, chicken, vegetable), 1 cup	10	Minestrone, ½ cup	50
Broth (beef, chicken), 1 cup	25	Oyster, clam, fish chowder, or stew (prepared with water), ½ cup	70
Broth (with rice or noodles), ½ cup	22	Tomato or vegetable, ½ cup	50
Consommé, clear, 1 cup	20		
"Cream of" soup (prepared with water), ½ cup	40		
Green pea soup, split pea, ½ cup	60	Any canned tomato or vegetable juice, 6-oz. glass	40